THE WONDER YEARS

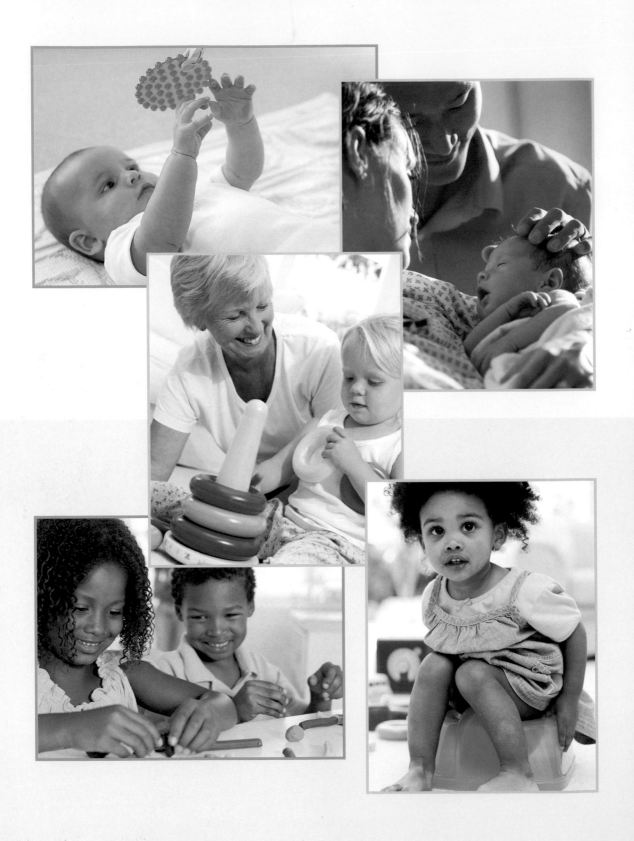

American Academy of Pediatrics

DEDICATED TO THE HEALTH OF ALL CHILDREN™

helping your baby and young child
successfully negotiate the major
developmental milestones

THE WONDER YEARS

Tanya Remer Altmann, MD, FAAP

EDITOR-IN-CHIEF

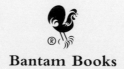

Bantam Books

THE WONDER YEARS
A Bantam Book / October 2006

Published by
Bantam Dell
A Division of Random House, Inc.
New York, New York.

Designed by: Emily Cook

Library of Congress Cataloging-in-Publication
Data is on file with the publisher

ISBN-10: 0-553-80476-6
ISBN-13: 978-0-553-80476-8

Printed and bound by Everbest in Hong Kong, China
Published simultaneously in Canada

www.bantamdell.com

10 9 8 7 6 5 4 3 2 1

The information contained in this publication should
not be used as a substitute for the medical care and
advice of your pediatrician. There may be variations
in treatment that your pediatrician may recommend
based on the individual facts and circumstances.
The information and advice contained in this book
apply equally to children of both sexes (except where
noted). To indicate this, we have chosen to alternate
between masculine and feminine pronouns
throughout the book.

contents

introduction

Congratulations! We assume that if you've bought this book or received it as a present, you've welcomed, or are about to welcome, a new son or daughter into your family. Your baby has spent the previous nine months developing in the uterus and has emerged as an infant with a limited number of reflex behaviors and an enormous desire and potential for acquiring skills in every area. It's now your "job" as parents to promote your baby's abilities and to help your baby achieve his or her full potential.

Helping your child to acquire the necessary developmental skills is a matter both of knowing what to expect and when, and what you can do to encourage emerging abilities. *The Wonder Years* has been created to enlighten parents about both these matters. It covers the normal processes of acquiring movement, fine motor, mental, social, and sensory skills as well as bowel and bladder control. It looks at personality and emotions, and how your baby begins to reason and think. It also shows, through a variety of fun-filled activities, how easy and enjoyable it is to promote these aspects of development, and it demonstrates how parents can create an environment in which their child can flourish physically, mentally, and emotionally.

First pictures
It's hard not to interpret this 31-week-old fetus' expression as a smile, though some scientists would say it's a reflex movement. At 12 weeks' gestation, this fetus not only is stepping on the surface of the uterus but he is able to bring his thumb to his mouth for sucking.

Your marvelous newborn

It was once thought that infants were like blank slates –
born into this world with minds free of all thought,
experience, and abilities. Ultrasound scanning and
fetology (the study of fetuses), among other scientific
disciplines, has shown this is not the case. We can
now see that babies put their thumbs into their
mouths to suck, reach for, and hold on to their
umbilical cords, "walk" on the surface of the womb,
and are capable of a great many facial expressions,
including yawns. These actions show that fetuses are
experimenting with touch sensations. Experiments
also prove that they recognize and respond to music
and other sounds. Today, doctors believe there is very
little that separates a fetus of around 35 weeks' gestation from a newborn.

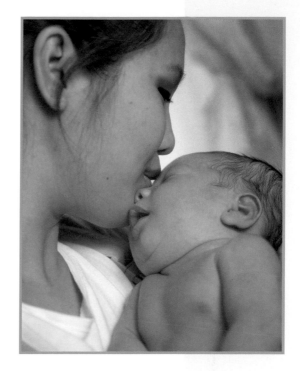

Sensory skills

Although it's not possible to measure things like eyesight and hearing in the
uterus, it is possible to do so with a newborn and it's now been proven that
babies are born with all their senses intact. As well as having a highly developed
sense of touch, babies can see and hear, distinguish between different tastes, and
have pronounced smell preferences.

Reflexes

Newborns also exhibit certain reflex behaviors (automatic physical responses
triggered involuntarily by a specific stimulus) that are important to survival. Many
of these remain in adulthood, such as the blink. Among the most important is the
rooting reflex. This requires a baby to turn his head automatically to any touch
on the cheek, and subsequent movements of his lips and tongue help him to take
the nipple into his mouth. The sucking and swallowing that follow are also
reflexes, as is gagging if he takes too much liquid in.

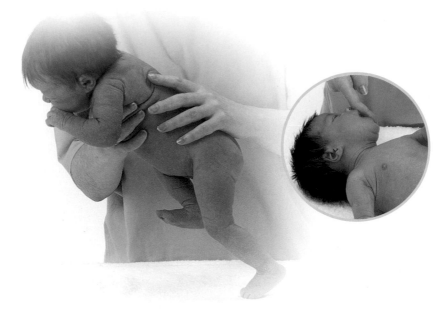

Rooting and walking
If you stroke a baby's cheek or the area around her mouth, she will turn her head in the direction of the stroking and may start to suck on your finger. If you hold your baby in a standing position on a flat surface, she will lift each foot in turn.

Other adaptive reflexes, such as the grasp reflex (if you place a finger across a baby's palm, he will close his fingers around it), may have been important in our evolutionary past but aren't helpful today. In fact, the persistence of the grasp reflex can impede a child acquiring manipulative skills. Some reflexes, like the Moro reflex (if the head is suddenly allowed to fall back a short way, the infant throws out his arms and extends his body) or walking (see above) are useful for diagnostic purposes – their presence or lack can reveal potential problems.

Other behavior

In addition to crying, your newborn can make a variety of noises. For example, he may hiccup a lot. This happens because the muscles that control breathing haven't perfected a steady rhythm. He also may sneeze frequently, which is generally due to light sensitivity rather than a respiratory problem, and he may sniffle, again not because he has a cold but because he has small nasal passages.

Generally, your baby will spend most of his time sleeping, although some babies are more wakeful than others. Crying is another common behavior. As you will learn, it is your newborn's primary means of communication, and it can mean a variety of things: That your baby is hungry, cold or hot, tired, lonely, or frightened.

The Wonder Years

The book's title reflects the fact that it is during the first five years of your child's life that he will develop from an infant, skilled only in primitive reflex behavior, into an individual who has mastered a wide range of physical activities, is dexterous, makes intelligent conversation, and is deemed ready to go to school. It is also during these years that you will often find yourself amazed and delighted by what and how quickly your baby learns.

To help you understand how your child masters a great variety of skills, the different aspects of development – movement, fine motor, sensory, mental, social and emotional, bowel and bladder control – are covered in individual chapters. Where some factor, such as play, is important to more than one area – in this case fine motor skills and social development – it is covered in both, with particular reference to specific aspects.

Each highly illustrated chapter starts with an overview of the approximate timing of events, and then covers in depth the major aspects of each skill. For example, in the fine motor skills chapter you'll discover how manipulation begins with reaching, grasping, and holding, and leads to picking up and letting go until a child is sufficiently mature to draw and cut and even dress himself. Throughout, Parental Participation features demonstrate activities that make the most of a baby's acquired skills, while a variety of boxes – Time for a Check-Up, Baby Booster, and In the know – provide important information on behavior and items that aid or impede development.

A number of special features throughout these chapters focus on providing experiences for your child that can help support the development of artistic, athletic, and social skills, as well as ensuring his safety.

Two further chapters – Developmental Concerns and Factors Affecting Development – contain important information on behavior and circumstances that can affect the normal course of development. Finally, there is a range of useful weight and height charts.

The American Academy of Pediatrics is dedicated to the well-being of all children. We hope that by reading this book you will become more aware and appreciative of your baby's potential to acquire skills and that you become better able to help him achieve his potential.

1

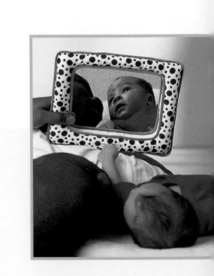

movement

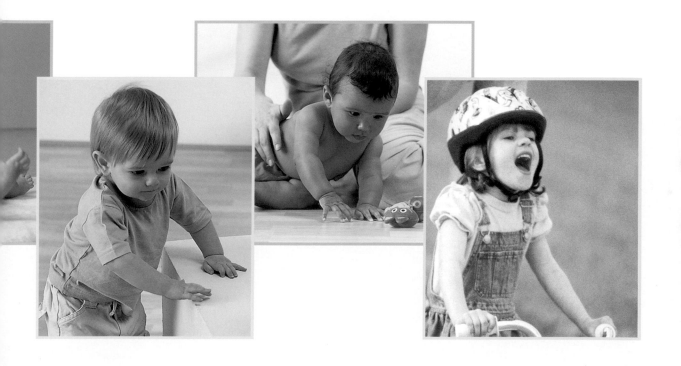

understanding the stages

Motor skills are those that require the coordinated movement of a muscle or a group of muscles. Gross motor movements are the large movements of the limbs and body, which are associated with crawling, running, and jumping. Initially, however, they are required to support your baby's body – enabling her to hold her head up steadily and sit without support – rather than moving it.

Gross motor skills depend on the strength of the large muscles that support and move the neck, back, arms, shoulders, and legs. In addition, the brain has to mature so that it is able to send the appropriate messages to these muscles. Fine motor skills also rely on muscle strength and messages from the brain but they produce more delicate movements, such as picking up a small object with the finger and thumb.

In early life, the parts of the brain that control and coordinate movement are immature. They gradually develop in a head-to-toe sequence, starting with the area responsible for controlling the movements of the head and neck, followed by the area that controls the movements of the arms and trunk, and finally the part that controls the movements of the legs. This sequence of development is illustrated in the milestones; head control is achieved before sitting, which is in turn learned before walking.

What happens
For a new skill to be learned, nerve pathways are laid down and the corresponding muscles are strengthened so that they can respond to the nerve impulses and produce the required movement. Motor skills are very complex; in addition to nerve pathways and muscle strength they require coordination of the muscles involved and balance. All of these are developed and reinforced through practice.

Both gross motor and fine motor skills develop throughout childhood; many activities require the two types of movements to occur at the same time.

The sequence of events
As with the other aspects of development, the stages of movement generally follow a recognized pattern, the achievement of one milestone forming the building block on which the next is built. The early movement milestones do not actually enable a baby to move from one place to another, but rather form the foundation for the more complex movements to come like rolling over and later walking. Achieving good head control, the first major movement milestone, is needed for all

other movements to occur. As with the other milestones, it is achieved through trying to do it again and again, but it can be helped along by the right environment and activities.

Aiding your child's progress

There are many things you can do to encourage gross motor achievements and share your child's joy as she progresses from rolling over for the first time to crawling, walking, and later running.

Look at the way your baby moves and find activities that use these movements. Vary the activities frequently as babies and toddlers have short attention spans.

Never push your child to learn but rather provide an environment that nurtures her development. Take her lead – she will soon let you know what she can manage and what needs to wait. Make her surroundings interesting and challenging, so that they encourage her to be active and to practice her skills. Always praise her efforts whether she succeeds or fails.

Seeking advice

As we have said before, every child is different and there can be a marked variation in the timing of the acquisition of skills from child to child. This variation is determined by a number of factors, two of the main ones being the time the parents achieved their milestones, and the opportunities given to practice a particular activity. Also, it is important to remember that premature babies tend to achieve their milestones later than full-term babies. In some cases, delayed learning can indicate an underlying problem. Always seek advice from your pediatrician if you have any

APPROXIMATE TIMING OF EVENTS	
The following are the ages around which your baby will achieve key developmental milestones.	
3 months:	Can be pulled to sitting with little or no head lag.
4 months:	Starts to roll from front to back.
4–5 months:	Acquires head control.
6 months:	Learns to roll from back to front. Sits supported.
6–8 months:	Sits unsupported for brief periods.
8 months:	Rolls over repeatedly.
9–11 months:	Pulls to standing for a few seconds before falling down. Learns to crawl.
11 months:	Sits down from standing – usually holding on to furniture. Starts to cruise around furniture and to walk with support.
11–12 months:	Starts to stand without support.
11–18 months:	Walks unaided.
12–15 months:	Starts to crawl upstairs.
14 months:	May learn to walk backward.
18 months:	Climbs into chairs and sits. Walks more steadily.
2 years:	Walks well. Can climb on and off furniture. Able to run. Climbs up and down stairs alone, with two feet per step.
3–4 years:	Goes up and down stairs alone, alternating feet.
4–5 years:	May be able to skip.

concerns. Remember, no one knows your child better than you do. Your child's pediatrician will be happy to see you and check that all is well with your little one.

head control

Gaining good head control is one of the major milestones of the first year and is needed for many key movements your baby will master from sitting unsupported to taking his first steps. The development of head control takes place gradually, but once accomplished will open up a whole new world to your baby.

Achieving good head control requires strengthening of the neck muscles that support and turn the head. Not only do babies need to learn how to support their heads when they are still, they also need to be able to alter the position of their heads frequently in response to what is happening around them and to hold their heads steady when they are moved, for example, when the car they are riding in goes around a corner. As with other milestones, they develop these skills through practice.

At the beginning

A newborn baby has weak muscles and his movements are uncontrolled, which means that his head needs to be carefully supported when he is moved. As well as having weak muscles, small babies have relatively large heads (about one-quarter of their length), which are heavy to support. When gently pulled to a sitting position, a newborn's head will lag behind. If you hold your young baby upright, his head may be upright momentarily before flopping forward onto your shoulder or back into your hand. If you place a small

Head lag
In the early months, when the neck muscles are weak, a baby's head will hang back when she is pulled to a sitting position, so always support your baby's head.

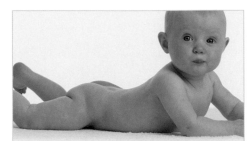

BABY BOOSTERS
PRONE POSITION

Babies who are frequently placed on their stomachs (prone position) often achieve head control earlier than those who spend most of their time lying on their backs. The AAP strongly recommends in their "Back to Sleep" campaign that babies always be put to sleep on their backs to reduce the risk of sudden infant death syndrome (SIDS). But when your baby is awake, if she spends time on her stomach, this will provide opportunities for her to learn to lift her head, a movement that strengthens the muscles of the neck and upper back. When lying prone, small babies naturally turn their heads to one side and soon start trying to lift their heads, probably as a result of their interest in what is going on around them. Therefore, it is very important to give your infant supervised time on her stomach during waking hours to encourage the development of head control.

baby on his stomach, he will turn his head to one side or the other as part of a natural response that ensures that he can continue to breathe.

The stages of head control

As in all aspects of development, the rate at which the various stages of head control are achieved varies from baby to baby. The following is therefore only a guide.

* *Around 1 month:* Your baby's head lags behind when he is pulled to a sitting position. When lying on his stomach, he may try to lift his head for a second.

* *Around 2 months:* If you hold your baby upright with your hands around his chest, he can hold his head up for a few seconds. Lying on his stomach, he can lift his head up to 45° for a few seconds.

* *Around 3 months:* By now, the head lag is less when your baby is pulled to a sitting position. When he sits supported, he may hold up his head for a few minutes. Lying on his stomach, he will lift up his head to 45° and even possibly 90°.

* *Around 4 months:* Your baby will lift his head and shoulders while resting on his hands and arms. When held in a sitting position, he has better head control but it is still a little wobbly. When lying on his back, he may lift his head briefly.

* *Around 5 months:* When held sitting, your baby's head is held up steadily and he can turn it from side to side. Lying on his stomach, he will lift his head and chest so that he can look straight ahead.

* *Around 6 months:* His neck muscles are very strong now and he can lift his head to look at his feet when lying on his back. Over the next few weeks, he will start to lift his head and look around.

PARENTAL PARTICIPATION

Children learn much of what they do through play. These simple activities will encourage your baby to look around and start to enjoy the world around him.

Mirror fun (from 1 month)

From an early age, a baby loves looking at himself, even though it will be some months before he knows who he is looking at! By 3 months he may begin to smile at his image. Turning to look in the mirror will help to increase the strength of his neck muscles and promote better head control. Hold an unbreakable mirror and look at it together.

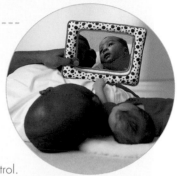

Tummy time (from 1 month)

Placing your baby on his tummy when he's awake will encourage him to lift his head. Begin by talking above his head. Within a few weeks, place a brightly colored toy in front of him to catch his attention.

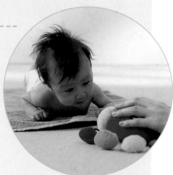

Bouncy bouncy (from about 5 months)

Once head control is achieved, your baby will love to play gentle bouncing games. Have him sit facing you, hold his hands and gently bounce him up and down while singing to him.

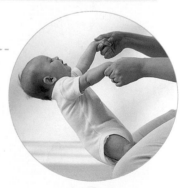

turning over

This is quite an achievement and is a baby's first experience of mobility; at first, she will delight in the sheer joy of moving – having spent weeks rooted in the same spot. Later, she will learn the skill of moving with a purpose – perhaps to get to toys that are out of her reach or to move toward you.

Babies usually start by rolling from front to back; it is easier to roll over from the prone (stomach) position than it is from the supine (lying on the back). The timing of many developmental milestones can be influenced by external factors and this is particularly the case with rolling onto the back. How early or late this happens will be determined to a great extent by the amount of time your baby spends lying on her stomach. Although babies should be placed on their backs to sleep, they should spend time on their stomachs when they are alert, not only to encourage the development of the neck and back muscles, but also to give them the chance to roll onto their backs. Lying on their stomachs, babies have the opportunity to see more of what is going on around them and being naturally inquisitive they make the most of this as soon as they can.

How turning over happens

From about three months of age, your baby will lift her head up to around 45° and then higher when lying on her stomach. Over the next few weeks, when lying on her stomach, she will learn to lift her head and chest off the floor, pushing up on her arms and arching her back. This gives her the opportunity to have a good look around. These mini push-ups are important for strengthening the muscles that will be needed when rolling over.

Quite often a baby will flip from her front to her back unintentionally – as a result of an involuntary shift in gravity as

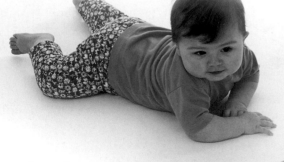

On a roll
This eight-month-old baby is adept at turning over in order to get a different view of her surroundings.

she pushes her chest off the ground. Using her arms as levers, she may shift her weight a little too far, which puts her off balance and she'll land on her back. And once she discovers what she can do, she will quickly try to repeat the action.

When it comes to rolling from back to front, however, this generally requires intention. Your baby must actively discover the actions that will tip her balance and propel her in the desired direction. This can take much practice and is fairly strenuous. Your baby needs to rock, roll, arch her body backward, twist one leg around and the other underneath in order to achieve a prone position.

Some babies are happy to spend weeks rocking to and fro without rolling over completely; others choose to roll in one direction and not the other, and some skip this milestone altogether and wait until they find another way of moving around, like crawling or scooting on their backs. The reason why this happens is not known but it is not a problem as long as your baby starts to show an interest in getting from one place to another.

The muscles developed for turning over are also important for subsequent milestones. Good head control as well as neck and upper back strength are needed to sit without support and to progress to crawling and later walking.

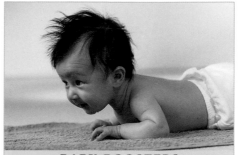

BABY BOOSTERS
SUPERVISED TUMMY TIME

Remember to lay your baby on his stomach when he is awake and alert. This will encourage him to lift up his head and chest. To further encourage your baby, sit in front of him holding a brightly colored toy. First hold it straight ahead and then later hold it a little higher so that he looks up. As he becomes able to lift his head higher and his chest off the floor, hold the toy a little higher and move it from side to side so that he must move his head to see it. This encourages him to look at objects as well as develop his movement skills.

! KEEP A HOLD
Babies may start to roll over around three months but this can happen earlier. For this reason, it is important never to leave your baby on a raised surface and to keep a hand on her at all times. Babies have no concept or fear of depth and do not perceive the danger of falling off a surface.

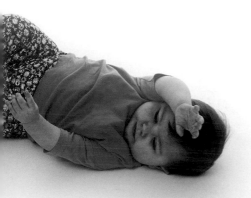

The stages of turning over

The skill of rolling over is usually acquired just before or around the same time as a baby starts to sit with a straight back (prior to this babies sit with a curved back). As with all developmental achievements, the timing of these stages varies between babies. As a guide:

* *Around 3 months:* At this age many babies start to turn over by rolling from their backs onto their sides and then onto their backs again. They will keep trying this until they eventually roll all the way over.

* *Around 4 months:* Your baby may now start to turn over from her stomach to her back. Some babies, however, roll from their backs to their stomachs first.

* *Around 6 months:* Your baby may now learn to roll from her back to her stomach. This is much harder than turning over from her stomach to her back. Her neck and arm muscles need to be very strong to make this happen.

* *Around 8 months:* Some babies now start to roll over repeatedly as a means of getting around. This can be great fun and forms the basis for many activities.

PARENTAL PARTICIPATION

Get rolling (from around 2½ months)

Around this age many babies are starting to build up toward their first roll. Try lying beside your baby and encouraging her to roll over toward you. Later (from 3 months), you also can place a colorful toy at her side but a little out of reach, so that she will eventually try to roll and get to it. Encourage your baby when she rolls by smiling, clapping, and praising her.

Roly poly (from around 6 months)

Once your baby can roll from her back to her front, it is time to play more floor games. Encourage her to roll over and over; also, once she is able to prop herself up on both arms, she will start to lean on only one arm and will be able to reach forward with the other for toys placed in front of her. Learning to reach one arm in front of her in this position is a first step in acquiring the skill of crawling.

sitting

Being able to sit gives a baby a different view of the world as well as the ability to play with a range of new and exciting toys. Most babies can sit unsupported by the age of eight months. The acquisition of this skill reflects the development taking place in the motor section of the brain and forms the basis for future movement.

The development of movement or motor skills starts with head control, which is achieved by strengthening of the muscles of the neck and upper back, and then moves down the body. As the muscles in the lower back become stronger and balance is acquired, a baby's ability to sit improves until he becomes able to sit unsupported. Within a few weeks, the muscles of his legs will develop and balance further improves so that crawling, standing, and later walking are achieved.

How sitting happens

Babies love to sit up and from as early as six weeks, a baby can sit supported in a baby chair. However, sitting babies for too long in their baby seats and strollers can mean they miss valuable opportunities to strengthen the muscles needed to sit alone and to improve their balance. Give your baby plenty of chances to sit with some support under your watchful eye.

Over the coming weeks, you will notice that your baby's back starts to straighten when he sits. He will learn to sit supporting himself with one or both hands placed on the floor and by about eight to nine months will be a proficient sitter. However, before this time, he'll often fall over as maintaining his balance while sitting is one of the hardest things he'll have to master. You may notice that your baby often wobbles for several seconds before he finds his balance and that he shifts his legs to steady himself.

Once he has acquired the skill to sit unsupported, he will learn to point to and reach forward for objects and to turn his head and twist his body to look at things. He now has a much wider visual range.

Reaching forward is an early stage of crawling; soon he will learn that he can support his body on all fours. Then it will only be a short time until he is on the move. It is time to think about child safety around your home (see page 28).

Looking out
While riding in the car, babies **must** face the rear in an infant-approved car safety seat positioned properly in the back seat. Never position his car seat in front of an airbag. When your baby is not in the car but still in his infant carrier, try facing him toward you to provide a more interesting view of his surroundings.

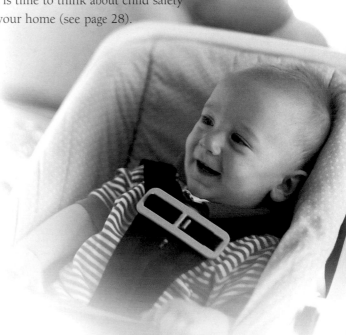

The average timing of the events that lead to sitting is:

* *Around 3 months:* Many babies can now be pulled to a sitting position with little or no head lag. Once held in a sitting position, the upper part of your baby's back is now straight, when previously the whole back was curved. However, the lower back continues to be curved for a few more weeks. Head control is now starting to emerge, with the head being held upright for brief periods.

* *Around 4 months:* Your baby may now be able to sit up as long as you support his arms. His back will now be straighter.

* *Around 6 months:* At this age, many babies can pull themselves to sitting when their hands are held. Once sitting with support, your baby will hold his head up and keep his back straight. He also will turn his head to see what's going on around him. Some babies may even sit unaided for a few seconds.

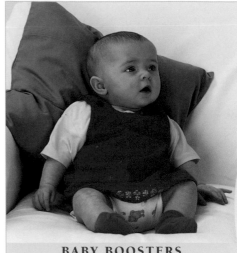

BABY BOOSTERS
SITTING WITH SUPPORT

Give your baby a chance to sit supported from around the age of two months – you can put her in a baby chair that will give her neck and back the support she needs. Alternatively you can prop her up with cushions but make sure they support her neck and back in a straight line. Mobiles hanging in her field of vision will amuse her. In addition, you can play clapping and singing games to catch her attention. Make sure your baby is supervised at all times.

Balanced sitting
To keep their bodies upright, babies have to find their center of gravity, which begins in the bottom and rises along the spine. Keeping the legs apart helps to widen this base and prevents toppling over.

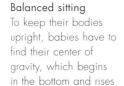

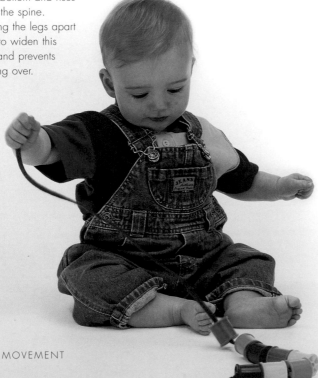

* *Around 6–8 months:* It is during this period that most babies learn to sit unsupported for longer periods. However, your baby can only sit still and will take a few more weeks to learn to reach out while keeping his balance.

* *Around 9 months:* Your baby will probably be able to sit on the floor amusing himself for longer periods now, although he may tire of sitting after 10 minutes or so. He will lean forward to reach objects but has yet to develop the skill of leaning sideways.

* **At 11 months:** Babies now start to sit down from standing with some control – at this stage they will usually hold on to furniture for support.

* **At 12 months:** Your baby will now be happy sitting for long periods, provided he has plenty to keep him amused. By now most babies learn to get into a sitting from a lying position.

* **By 15 months:** Your baby will have learned to lie down from sitting.

* **At 15–18 months:** Babies learn to climb into adult chairs and sit.

Time to eat

The AAP believes that breastfeeding is the optimal source of nutrition through the first year of life. When your baby seems curious about foods that others are eating, can push food from the front toward the back of his mouth with his tongue, and is able to sit supported for a time, he may be ready for solid foods to be introduced. High chairs allow babies to take part in family meals and are a great vantage point to see what's happening; they also give babies the chance to sit supported while playing with small toys on the food table.

STRAP HIM IN

Although most babies are quite stable sitting on the floor by about eight months, it is important to remember that your baby can still topple over and he should only sit on chairs with straps. He also should continue to be strapped into his stroller and car safety seat. **Always** supervise your baby.

Activities that strengthen the neck and upper back muscles also will prepare your baby for sitting. Once your baby can sit with and then without support, you can have all sorts of fun together.

Sitting play
(from around 6 months)

You can sit your baby on the floor surrounded by cushions to soften his fall if he topples over. Give him safe, interesting objects to play with. Never leave your baby sitting alone, even with support, as he may topple face down into a cushion and be unable to push himself up. You also can sit cross-legged and sit your baby with his bottom against your legs for support.

Sitting together
(from around 9 months)

Your baby will enjoy sitting on the floor with you for longer periods, playing with toys, singing, or clapping together.

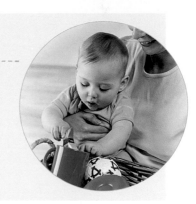

In the big bath (from around 6 months)

Once your baby can sit alone or with only a little support, he is ready to sit in the bath. This can be a source of great fun – let him splash; give him bath toys as well as cups and other containers for pouring. Never leave your baby alone – even for a moment – in the bathtub. Infant bath seats or support devices are not a substitute for caregiver supervision.

crawling

There will be big changes when your baby starts to crawl. Your baby will love the newfound freedom she gets from being on the move but your life will become more challenging. You cannot leave your baby lying happily on her mat even for a moment while you dash to get something – there will be no way of knowing where she will be when you come back! On the other hand, you and your baby will have great fun together while she explores her surroundings.

As well as developing her gross motor skills, learning to crawl will give your baby the opportunity to pick up, examine, and put down interesting objects, so improving her fine motor skills. She also will use her visual skills as her perspective develops and the world becomes a three-dimensional place.

As your baby learns to crawl, her coordination improves and she strengthens the muscles she will soon use for cruising and later for walking unsupported. The average age for learning to crawl is about nine months. It usually happens when a baby can sit up steadily; this shows that her neck and back muscles are strong and that her sense of balance is developing well. However, there is a good deal of variation in the timing of learning to crawl

and, in fact, some babies never crawl at all, but find other ways of getting around. These include wiggling on their tummies and rolling and scooting on their backs (they may use one hand and one buttock

> ### CAUTION
> Now that your baby can get around, it is important to keep potentially harmful objects and substances out of her way. Babies also learn to climb up the stairs within a few weeks of starting to crawl; stair gates at the top and bottom of the stairs will prevent tumbles from climbing up or down unsupervised.

Interlimb interaction
Most babies who crawl on all fours alternate between moving opposite hands and knees – their left hands with their right knees and their right hands with their left knees.

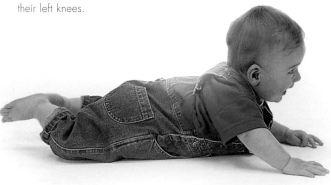

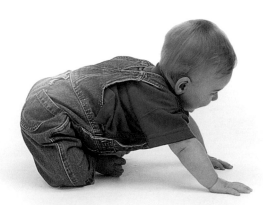

or both hands and both buttocks), or move along on all fours (sometimes known as bear-walking). Babies choose the most energy efficient ways of getting around. Some babies learn to pull themselves up to standing and then to cruise very early, skipping the early ways of getting around altogether or using them only briefly. Whether babies crawl or not does not seem to influence when they start to walk; babies who crawl tend to start walking around the same time as those who never crawl.

The stages of crawling

From birth, babies are developing skills that will equip them for learning to crawl and later walk. Around six months, your baby will begin to acquire key skills:

* **At 6 months:** Most babies can now lift their heads, chests, and abdomens off the floor when lying on their stomachs. They support themselves with straight arms and place their palms flat on the floor.

* **At 7 months:** Your baby will now probably be able to support herself in the crawling position with only one hand. This allows her other hand to reach forward as it will when she crawls.

* **At 8 months:** Your baby may get into a crawling position and then rock backward

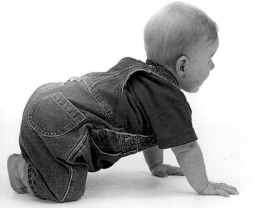

TIME FOR A CHECK-UP

It is always important to remember that all babies are different and acquire their skills at their own pace. However, by the age of one, most babies are on the move whether it be by crawling, scooting, or in some cases, walking. If this has not happened, it is important to talk to your pediatrician, who will examine your baby to check that all is well.

and forward as if revving up before she finally pushes off. Holding her in a standing position on your knee so that she can straighten her legs will help to build up the leg muscles she needs. Within a few weeks she will learn that the way to get around is to advance one hand and the leg on the opposite side at the same time.

* **At 9 months:** Babies of this age may wiggle on their tummies and some start to crawl. Often babies crawl backward first. Because their arm muscles are stronger than their leg muscles some babies find it easier to push backward rather than forward. Initially their tummies may still touch the floor. If your baby is a proficient backward crawler, it may take a chance discovery to get her crawling forward.

* **At 11 months:** Your baby may now be able to crawl on her hands and knees with her tummy clearing the floor. She is now really on the move and will pick up speed as she gains experience and confidence. At first she will plunge headfirst over steep slopes and across wide gaps, but with time her judgment will improve and her movements will become more controlled. Many babies continue to crawl for some months, after they have started walking, particularly when they want to get somewhere quickly.

PARENTAL PARTICIPATION

There are many things you can do with your baby that will encourage her to get moving, therefore improving her coordination and building up her muscles.

Making a tunnel

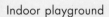

Once your baby learns to crawl, she will love getting through things. You can make a simple tunnel by draping a tablecloth over a table or wide-legged chair. Put interesting toys inside the tunnel for your baby to retrieve.

Indoor playground

You can turn your living room into an exciting obstacle course for your baby by placing cushions and boxes on the floor for her to navigate around. You can also encourage her to keep moving by placing toys and other objects out of her reach.

Catch me if you can (from around 6 months)

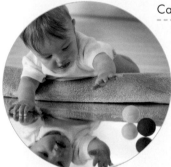

Babies of this age love following brightly colored rolling toys. Not only do these encourage them to crawl, they also improve hand-eye coordination when they try to reach out for them. Placing a mirror underneath some balls will provide extra interest; while a rolled-up towel placed for your baby to crawl over encourages an up-and-over movement.

Up and over (from around 10 months)

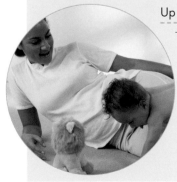

This will encourage your baby to get moving. Lie on your side with your baby behind you and place a toy in front of you. Encourage her to climb over you to reach the toy.

standing and cruising

So far, all your baby's ways of getting around, whether they be crawling, scooting, or rolling, have kept his hands occupied, which has limited some of his other activities. By learning to stand and later walk, he will be freeing up his hands and widening his choices of entertainment.

From nine months, or earlier, your baby will probably learn to pull himself to a standing position. For some time he will continue to need support, either from you or from nearby objects and furniture. He is working his way to his ultimate aim – to walk unaided. This will enable him to move more quickly and to pick up anything interesting he encounters.

To pull themselves to standing, babies need to have the basic requirements – head control and strong back muscles. They also need strong leg muscles, including those around the hips, as well as strong arms. A baby's legs are short in comparison to the rest of his body and to support the upper torso requires determination as well as muscular power and coordination. Balance is crucial to standing unsupported and it takes several weeks for this to develop.

Within a few weeks of standing, your baby will learn to move first one and then the other foot.

Before your baby walks unsupported, he will side step using furniture and other objects for support. He will move along the furniture by sliding his hands along while at the same time moving his first foot along the ground and then sliding his second foot along to meet it. This is

known as cruising and tends to start around the age of 11 or 12 months.

Cruising will exercise your baby's brain. He will need to decide how to get across gaps and, in doing so, will consider a number of options. He will also find out something about his size in relation to other things.

The timing of events

As with all developmental milestones, the timing of learning to stand and cruise varies, but the sequence of events is similar and acquiring one skill gives a baby the basis for learning the next. In some cases,

Bow legs
Most babies have bow legs when they are learning to stand and walk. This is perfectly normal and will resolve over the next 12 months or so.

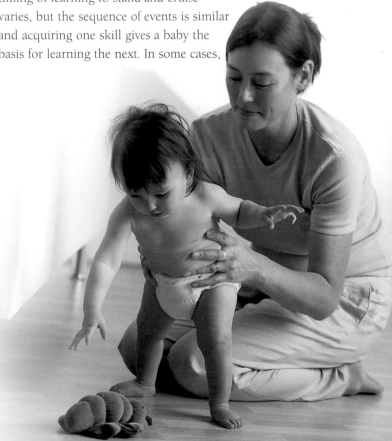

however, crawling or other early ways of getting around may be missed out. The average timing of events is:

* *At 9 months:* Your baby may learn to pull himself up to stand. He will stay on his feet for a few seconds while he holds on to something for support. He will then fall down onto his bottom with a thud. Initially, this may be a shock for him, but soon he may find falling down on his bottom fun. Over the next few weeks, his muscle strength, balance, and coordination will increase until he is able to stand alone.

You can help your baby by teaching him to sit down from standing. Gently bend your baby's knees and holding both his hands, lower him slowly until his bottom reaches the ground.

* *At 11 months:* Your baby may start to cruise around furniture at this age. Some babies stand alone for a few moments and some may walk with support. Some may even begin to walk unaided. At first babies

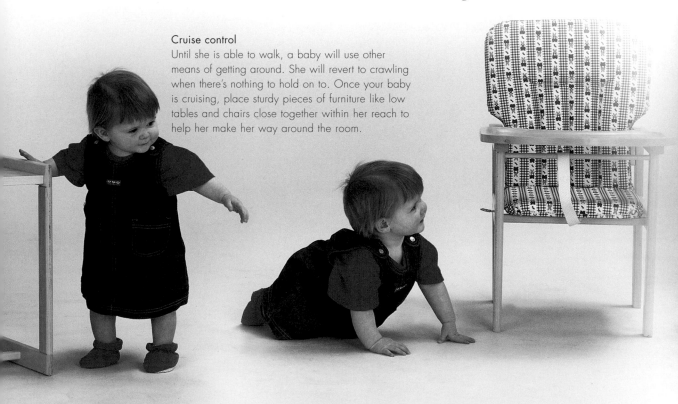

Cruise control
Until she is able to walk, a baby will use other means of getting around. She will revert to crawling when there's nothing to hold on to. Once your baby is cruising, place sturdy pieces of furniture like low tables and chairs close together within her reach to help her make her way around the room.

need to slide their hands along furniture when they are cruising, but soon they will let go with one hand enabling them to get hold of the next piece of furniture. A key stage in learning to walk is when babies start to lift their feet in turn rather than sliding them along; this means that for a brief moment they are standing on one leg – a major achievement.

✳ *From 12 months:* Babies start to stand without support around one year of age. This gives them the chance to start to play with a whole new selection of toys that were previously out of reach. As your baby learns to walk, the world will become a much bigger place and he will enjoy his independence as he starts to explore it.

✳ *At 14 months:* Many babies can stand alone for longer periods at this age. They can bend over and stand back up again, while still maintaining their balance.

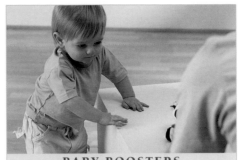

BABY BOOSTERS
TEMPTING TOYS

Putting a toy on a low table will encourage a baby to pull himself to standing to reach it. Once a baby can stand with little support, a low table with interesting objects on it can provide the support necessary while encouraging him to use his hands. Try colorful plastic cups or building blocks. When he is ready, encourage him to stand alone by holding his hands and then slowly letting go – he'll soon let you know if he is not ready. Be ready to catch him if he falls!

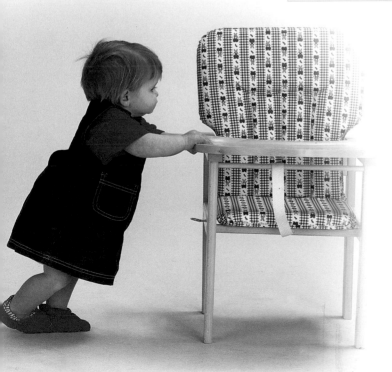

MAKE IT SAFE

In the early stages of standing up and cruising, babies can easily tumble over. This is part of the learning process. The important thing is to make the environment they fall in as safe as possible while still allowing them to test themselves and develop their skills. Sharp corners on furniture should be covered with padding and babies should be protected from other hazards like fireplaces. You also need to ensure that all the furniture is stable so that your baby can rely on it for support.

keeping your child safe

Young children are naturally curious. They learn about the world by physically interacting with the objects around them. They like to touch, feel, and explore. They also learn about properties of things by putting them in their mouths. But indulging your child's innate interest carries risk. Most children under the age of five have very little sense of danger – they are unaware of hazards and will inadvertently place themselves at risk in order to go wherever their curiosity leads them. Very young children will drink anything, be attracted to moving objects and objects that make interesting noises, and crawl into small spaces. And, because they are just beginning to learn to control their bodies, they can easily trip or fall. As a result, they are at high risk for injuries due to choking, drowning, poisoning, and fires. This natural tendency to explore the world around them, combined with their inability to recognize danger and to inhibit their actions, can put young children at high risk of injury. Here are some tips for ensuring that your child can exercise her curiosity safely.

Childproof your home

Do your best to ensure that your home is safe for your curious learner. Install electrical outlet covers, window guards, gates at the top and bottom of the stairs, smoke and carbon monoxide detectors, and barriers around fireplaces or other heat sources.

Put strong locks on cupboard doors to stop her from getting inside and taking medicines, cleaning products, or cosmetics.

Keep knives and electrical appliances out of reach, and make sure the cords are not accessible.

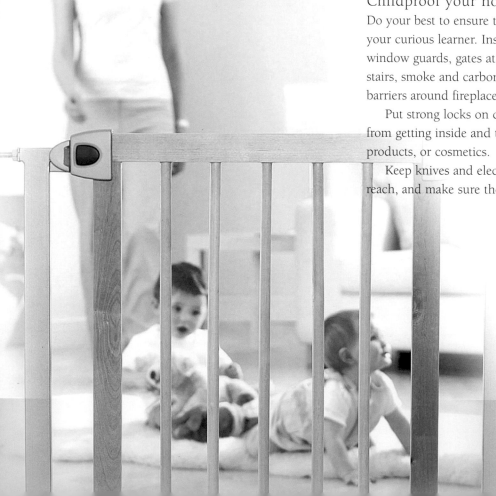

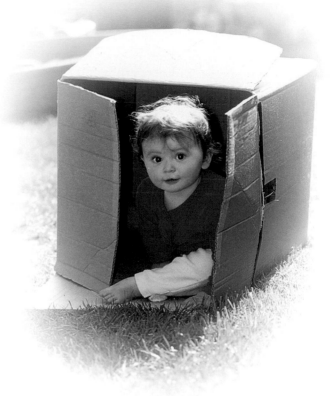

Set limits

Make sure some are positive as well as negative. Tell your toddler what she can and cannot do, so that she knows where she can explore as well as knows which areas are off-limits. Try to have more "do" rules than "don't" rules.

Help her explore safely

Your child has a natural need to explore, no matter how much you try to restrict her. As she gets older, and as appropriate, teach her how to play without putting herself at risk rather than trying to confine her to specific parts of the house. For example, teach her never to pick and eat anything from a plant when she goes into the yard, and that she is not to put her face too close to an animal.

Be protective but allow safe fun

Your child won't learn without actively engaging with the world around her, and that always involves some degree of risk. Encourage her to try new activities and explore, but always ensure that your child is properly equipped. Make sure, for example, that she wears appropriate protective gear such as a helmet when riding a tricycle or bike, and that she doesn't play on playground equipment with dangling shoelaces, or drawstrings on a jacket or shirt.

SIMPLE-TO-INSTALL CHILD SAFETY DEVICES

- Safety latches and locks keep the contents of cabinets and drawers out of reach of children.
- Safety gates prevent children from entering dangerous areas and falling downstairs.
- Doorknob covers and door locks stop children from entering rooms unsupervised.
- Doorstops and door holders protect fingers and hands from injury.
- Window guards and safety barriers prevent falls from windows, balconies, decks, and landings.
- Outlet covers and plates help prevent electrocution.

stepping and walking

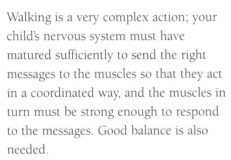

Walking is a key developmental milestone and a sign that your baby is progressing well along the road to independence. He may take his first steps around 12 months and will quickly learn to walk unaided and later to run, jump, and skip. With all milestones, there is variation in the time they begin to be achieved but this is particularly the case with walking. Often, late walking runs in the family but in some cases, a delay in learning to walk reflects an underlying problem.

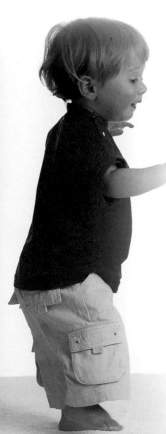

Steady as he goes
Babies begin walking with their arms held out for balance, their legs spread wide apart, and their feet turned outward.

Walking is a very complex action; your child's nervous system must have matured sufficiently to send the right messages to the muscles so that they act in a coordinated way, and the muscles in turn must be strong enough to respond to the messages. Good balance is also needed.

It is not possible to get a child walking before he is ready. However, you can provide a suitable environment by giving your child plenty of praise and making his surroundings stimulating to encourage him to get moving.

Once a baby can walk he has more opportunities to explore his surroundings and to examine what he finds. He will begin to plan sequences of actions; at first they will be simple, like crossing the room to pick up a toy and then coming back to where he was.

The timing of events
Throughout a baby's first year, he is gradually strengthening the muscles he needs for one of his greatest achievements so far – taking his first steps. At around nine months, he may pull himself to a

TIME FOR A CHECK-UP
As we have already said, there is great variation in when babies learn to walk. The important thing is that they make progress – a baby who achieves other movement milestones, like good head control and crawling late is likely to walk late but the skills should be achieved within a reasonable timeframe. If your baby has not walked by the time he is 18 months, talk to your pediatrician. He or she will evaluate all the aspects of your child's development, whether your baby can sit unsupported, roll over, crawl, pull himself to standing, and cruise around furniture. Your pediatrician will also assess your child's development with regards to walking at his 15- and 18-month exams. In most cases of delayed walking, the findings will be normal but sometimes tests will be arranged to exclude an underlying disorder.

stand and then it is only a matter of a few months before he will take this great step toward independence. Most babies learn to walk at around 13 months. A few may walk as early as 11 months. Do not worry if your child takes longer to find his feet; many children do not learn to walk until they are 16 or 17 months – as long as they are otherwise developing normally, this is not usually a problem. On average, the stages of walking occur at around these times:

✴ *At 11 months:* Most babies start to cruise at around this time, taking sideways steps around furniture. At first, items of furniture need to be no more than an arm's length apart. Gradually, babies learn to move along furniture that is farther apart, meaning they are able to walk alone very briefly.

Many 11 month olds will walk with one or both arms held or pushing a sturdy push toy. They may also stand alone for a few moments.

✴ *At 12 months:* Some babies may walk alone.

✴ *At 14 months:* Your baby may now be learning to walk backward.

✴ *At 15 months:* Many babies walk alone by this age but they still tend to be a little unsteady, keeping their feet wide apart and arms out to help them balance. They also need to learn how to stop in a controlled way; they may still bump into things frequently. Your baby will probably enjoy playing with pull-along and push-along toys now.

✴ *At 18 months:* Your baby will probably be walking more steadily now; his legs will be closer together and he will be able to stop more easily; he will not need to hold his arms out anymore to balance. He will

PARENTAL PARTICIPATION

Walking unaided takes a good deal of confidence. You can help your baby on his way by giving him plenty of praise and also with the following activities.

Walking together

Take the time to walk with your baby whenever possible; it is all too easy to put him in the stroller when you want to get somewhere. He will really appreciate and benefit from time on his feet. At first he will need to hold both of your hands, then one hand and then perhaps just one finger. Eventually, he will be ready to walk alone – let him do this in his own time. Do not suddenly let go of his hand before he is ready. Once he is ready to go, stand a short distance away from him and encourage him to come toward you.

Get dancing

Toddlers love moving around to music. Play different types of music for your baby – slow, fast, and different styles. Dance with your toddler – she will love it!

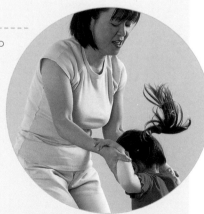

start to speed up and may even be able to run in his own toddler way.

✻ From around 2 years: Toddlers are expert walkers by now and have acquired the skill of walking heel to toe just as adults do.

In the know... *Baby walkers*

The AAP recommends against the use of mobile baby walkers, because they are dangerous and associated with many injuries. In addition, they may give babies too much support and therefore slow the acquisition of balance and the muscle strength needed in the legs for walking. Recent research has shown that using baby walkers can be associated with delayed onset of independent walking. Your baby still needs plenty of opportunity to walk barefoot. This will give him a greater sense of stability as it brings his feet into closer contact with the walking surface and allows him to adjust the position of his feet easily.

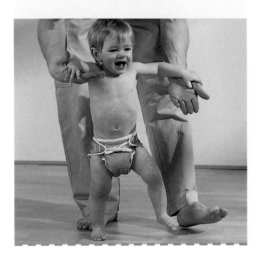

Reasons for late walking

There may be various reasons why a baby's walking is late.

✻ A common cause is delay in maturation of the nerves and muscles involved in walking; often this is a normal delay that runs in a family. In such cases, other aspects of development will be normal and movement skills will also be normal but delayed. The child's development will be carefully monitored.

✻ Some babies find they can get around quickly and efficiently by scooting or crawling and so have no real incentive to start walking.

✻ A lack of opportunity to practice walking may be a factor for some children; an example of this would be a child who has been ill and confined to bed for a prolonged period. Also, in some cases, overprotective parents limit what their baby does and so their chances to learn to walk.

✻ In some cases, late walking reflects learning disabilities or developmental delay.

✻ In some cases, delayed walking results from one of a number of disorders that affect the muscles, or, as in cerebral palsy, where there is damage to the developing brain.

It is important to remember to schedule regular physical exams with your child's pediatrician so that he or she can follow your child's development.

kneeling and climbing

Throughout childhood, but particularly in their early years, children build on their achievements rapidly to make life more exciting. They love climbing and will seize any opportunity to get off the ground. Your baby may start to crawl up stairs between the ages of 12 and 15 months. By 18 months, she will probably be climbing whenever she can. When she climbs into a chair, she may enter it facing backward and then turn around to sit facing the right way.

Children also learn to kneel at about 15 months. At first they will need support, but by 18 months most children can kneel unaided. To help your child perfect her kneeling skills, when she's bent down, offer her some toys. Unless she is very good at balancing, she may want to hold on to a secure support surface such as a coffee table.

At 18 months, toddlers enjoy climbing around on the furniture. However, they can fall off easily and so need close supervision. Now is the time your child can start to play on low climbing apparatus, again under your watchful eye. Toddlers of this age are constantly testing themselves – and your nerves! It is important to strike the balance between creating a safe environment while allowing your child to develop her skills and confidence.

Perfecting skills

Rapid advances in climbing and walking take place from year two to three.

✳ From around 2 years: Many toddlers can climb onto furniture and then climb down again. Your child may get up onto a sofa or chair to look out of the window and may climb up to get a toy that is out of her reach. For some time, she will climb down backward reaching her feet out until they feel the floor beneath her.

Also, around the time of her second birthday, your child will begin to refine her walking skills, learning how to stop, change direction, speed up, and slow down without landing on her bottom. She also will become better at balancing and her gait will become steadier.

✳ By 2½ years: Children are able to climb on simple play equipment with confidence and will really start to enjoy climbing structures and slides.

Stair climbing
Climbing upstairs is easier than climbing down. Your child may "get stuck" on his way down. At just over two years, your child will walk down one step at a time, with both feet on each step. After three years they start to alternate feet.

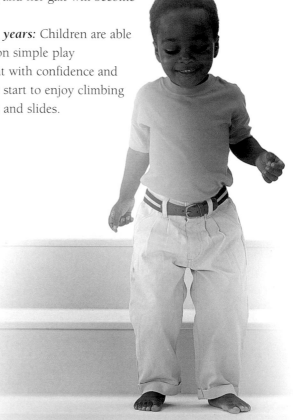

✳ *From around 3 years:* Children are becoming very agile and will be able to make the most of visits to the playground. This agility will continue to develop with many four year olds being able to climb trees and longer ladders skillfully.

Getting up and down stairs

Babies may start to make their way upstairs from as early as 12 months, well before they walk competently. At first, a baby will use a mixture of crawling and walking to go upstairs and will usually come downstairs by sliding down feet first on her tummy – this tends to start between the ages of 12 and 15 months.

Between 18 months and two years, a toddler will move up a step at a time, using one knee to lead the way and support her body as she brings up her opposite leg. If you help her to walk upstairs, she will put one foot on the step and then bring the other up to meet it rather than walking up the stairs

individually. From the age of two years or so, a toddler may walk up with her hand against the wall for support, but will still have two feet on each step. She will first come downstairs by creeping down backward or scooting down on her bottom – many toddlers find this a great game. Your child will then progress to walking downstairs on her feet, again with two feet on each step, but will need to hold a hand for support. It is only after age three that children begin alternating feet on each step as they first master going up stairs and later down.

Install safety gates at the top and bottom of the stairs to prevent serious injury and to help ensure that your child does not try to sneak up or down stairs unsupervised.

The great escape

Your child may start to climb out of her crib at around 18 months – or earlier. As soon as she can pull to a stand, remove

Problem solving
Starting at around 15 months, toddlers become accomplished and creative climbers. They will enter a chair facing backward and end up sitting forward.

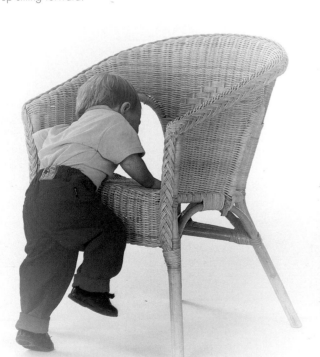
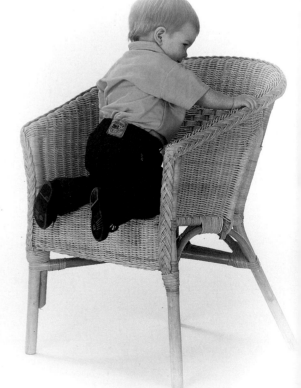

any bumper pads that could be used as steps for climbing out. Set the mattress to its lowest point before she can stand, and when she is 35 inches tall or the side rail is less than three-quarters of her height, move her to a bed. To prevent the most serious of falls, make sure to never place your child's crib or bed near a window.

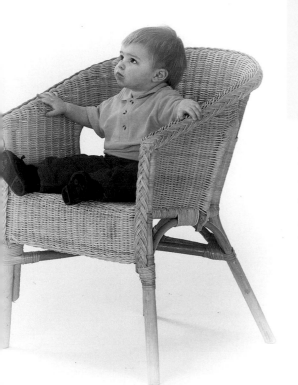

PARENTAL PARTICIPATION

Playground equipment can entertain your child for many years. To prevent injuries, make sure the equipment and surfaces are safe and closely supervise your child during play.

Slides

Teach your child to use the ladder to climb up to the sliding surface and to walk away from the bottom of the slide as soon as she reaches it. If a slide has been in the sun, check before use to make sure it is not hot.

Swings

Swing seats should be made of a soft and flexible material. Teach your child never to share the same swing or to walk in front of or behind a swing while another child is playing on it.

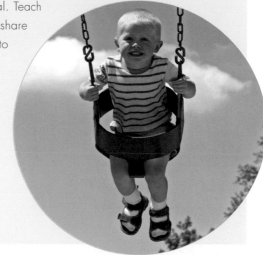

Playground surfaces

Concrete, asphalt, packed earth, and grass surfaces aren't safe for use under playground equipment. Safer examples include wood chips or mulch (at least 9 inches deep for equipment up to 7 feet high) and sand (at least 9 inches deep for equipment up to 5 feet high). Frequent maintenance of these surfaces is very important to assure protection in case of falls.

activity for young children

Exercise has many benefits – it strengthens muscles as well as improving coordination and balance. Young children naturally want to be active and as a parent it is important to promote safe, free-play activities. Children who get plenty of physical activity are likely to be happier and to sleep better. Encouraging children to exercise early in life will set a pattern for a healthy lifestyle in the future.

Baby games
Even babies from as young as six weeks can benefit from some gentle activity.

* *Hands up:* Lay your baby on his back and let him get hold of your forefingers or thumbs. Then gently alternate raising one arm and then the other over his head.
* *Cycling fun:* Hold his ankles, and rotate his legs as if cycling – go one way and then the other.
* *Cross your heart:* Hold his hands and gently open his arms wide and bring them across his chest.

Infant exercise
This is a fun way for small children to use their movement skills through a series of gentle exercises and games. Although baby and preschool exercise classes are readily available in many areas, opportunities for supervised, unstructured, and explorative activities in a safe environment will benefit your infant (and toddler) more.

Swimming
Learning to swim is very important from a safety point of view and can provide great exercise for older children. Although infant and toddler aquatic classes are popular and provide enjoyment for parents and caregivers, children are generally not ready for formal swimming lessons until after the age of four. Drowning is a leading cause of injury and death in children. Having children begin swimming lessons at an earlier age does not lead to

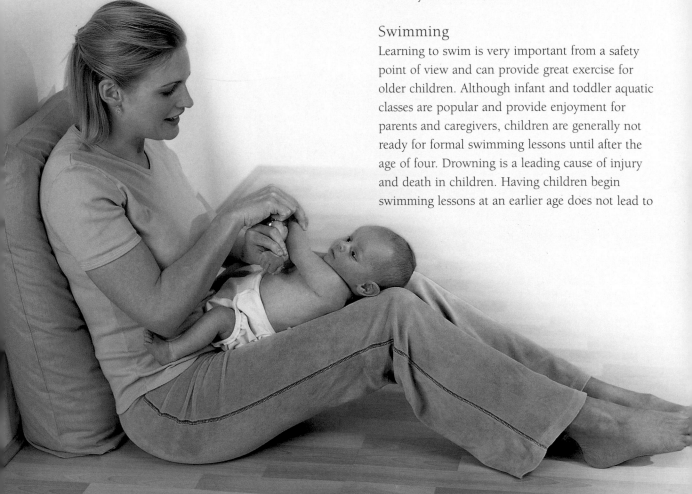

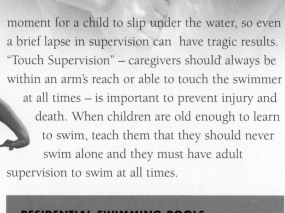

CAUTION

Never leave babies and young children unsupervised in or near water, even when it is very shallow. Even young children who demonstrate an ability to swim need to be closely watched and kept in "Touch Supervision" at all times.

mastery of swim skills or water safety sooner compared with those children who start swim lessons at a later age.

Regardless of an infant's or toddler's apparent level of comfort and competence in or around the water, constant close supervision by an adult is necessary to prevent drowning. It only takes a

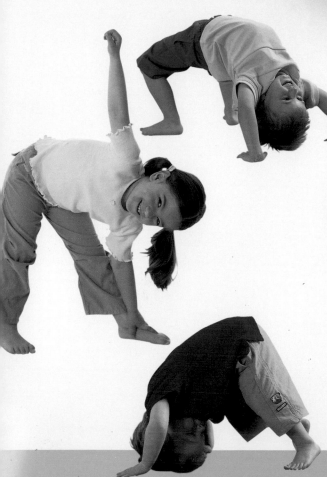

moment for a child to slip under the water, so even a brief lapse in supervision can have tragic results. "Touch Supervision" – caregivers should always be within an arm's reach or able to touch the swimmer at all times – is important to prevent injury and death. When children are old enough to learn to swim, teach them that they should never swim alone and they must have adult supervision to swim at all times.

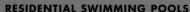

RESIDENTIAL SWIMMING POOLS

- Is there a four-sided fence at least 4 feet high with a self-closing and self-latching gate surrounding your pool?
- Do all caregivers know CPR?
- Is there a telephone and rescue equipment (e.g. life preservers, life jackets, shepherd's crook) nearby in case of emergency?

running, jumping, and skipping

Once she's learned to walk, your child will keep on making great strides in terms of balance and agility. By the time she is three, she will have mastered many active movements and will be able to perform them without a second thought. Over the coming years, her choice of physical activities and games will rapidly increase as her skills develop.

On the run

Most children begin to run between 18 months and two years of age. At first, they look at the ground about two yards in front of them all the time. They can manage with running straight ahead but may have problems when things get in their way, which means they need to change direction suddenly.

* *Around 2 years:* Your child will be running more easily. She will put her whole foot down and over the next year or so she will learn to start, stop, and run around obstacles. By the age of four, many children can run up and down stairs. They move around with skillful ease and by five can run on their toes, enabling them to be even more agile and to change direction frequently.

A hop, skip, and a jump

Children learn to jump during their third year, usually at the age of two and a half or so. They may start by jumping from a low step with their feet together; they will also jump on the ground, again with their feet together. At first, your child will want to hold your hand for support but before too long she will be happy to do it alone.

* *By 3 years:* Children can jump from the bottom step. They can also stand for a very short time on one foot. This indicates their balancing skills are developing well and is the forerunner to learning to hop.

* *At 4 years:* Your child can balance on one foot for up to five seconds. Children also learn to hop at this stage; they usually prefer one particular foot over the other.

* *At 5 years:* Children have really honed their motor skills. They can balance on

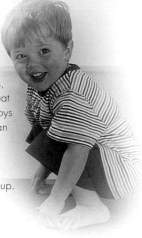

Squatting down

At around two years, children learn to squat down to play with toys on the floor. They can stand up from a squatting position without using their hands to push them up.

one leg for up to 10 seconds and can hop 10 times in a row. They also can skip on alternate feet. All these activities illustrate the excellent balancing skills that have been developed by this age.

Top activities

By the age of four your child will probably enjoy playing a simple version of hopscotch. Don't worry about the numbers too much; focus on jumping around and having fun. Draw out the squares and let her enjoy jumping and hopping from one to another. You can play, too! As she learns her numbers and her agility improves, she will enjoy playing the traditional game with her friends.

Your child also might like to try a simple variation of the game Twister, where she will have to move her hands and feet onto different colored circles. You can make a variation by putting colored paper on the floor and calling out colors.

A good way to exercise all your child's abilities is to ask her to imitate various animals; she'll oblige by jumping like a bunny, squatting like a frog, slithering like a snake, or leaping like a kangaroo.

PARENTAL PARTICIPATION

Musical and movement games can be part of playdates or parties. Children as young as 18 months love moving to music. By the time your child is about three years old, she will be able to play simple musical games. Make sure your child has a chance to calm down and catch her breath after running around.

Musical games and "Freeze Dance"

The children either dance around until the music stops and then sit down or freeze. Strictly speaking the last to sit down or the one who moves is out, but young children will be happy to keep playing without a winner.

Traffic lights "Stop and Go"

One person (adult or child) stands at the front and gives the instructions – "Green light" run around; "Yellow light" slow down; "Red light" stop; "Traffic jam" walk slowly. Younger children will simply enjoy following the instructions and running around; there is no need to have a winner. With older children, anyone doing the wrong action may be called out.

Follow the leader

One person leads around the room and the others follow in a line and copy the actions. If an adult is the leader they can vary the actions and make the game more fun.

Music and movement

Select some gentle, restful music and ask the children to pretend to be trees blowing in the wind, a kite in the sky, or a cat going to sleep.

sport skills

At age five, your child will be well on the way to mastering all the basic skills involved in movement but he will go on refining them and integrating them into more complex movement sequences. For example, a five-year-old can both run and kick a ball but not do both well at the same time.

Bike time
Riding around not only gives your child a chance to expend energy but she also will be acquiring vital coordination skills.

From an early age, when movement skills are developing rapidly, encourage your child to engage in free-play activities on a regular basis, especially outdoors. Fostering a love for outdoor exercise can help children develop active lifestyles. Your pediatrician can help suggest a sport or activity appropriate for your child. Around six years of age, most children are ready for organized team sports such as soccer or softball. Remember, the early appearance or development of a specific sport skill does not necessarily predict future success in that

sport. What's important is to help your child find a sport he enjoys and be a role model by participating in activity as well.

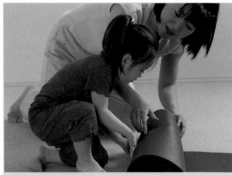

BABY BOOSTERS
ENCOURAGING ACTIVITY

Obesity is increasing rapidly in children. Regular exercise combined with a balanced diet can prevent this serious and potentially life-threatening problem. Regular exercise in childhood also reduces the risk of developing serious medical conditions such as joint problems and heart disease in adulthood. It also helps to elevate mood and improve general well-being.

As well as encouraging your child to exercise and run around with her friends, make exercise and being active a way of life for your family.

Cycling

Although most children lack the balancing skills necessary for riding a two-wheeler until the age of seven or eight, young toddlers can prepare to ride a bicycle by playing on stationary toys and older ones will enjoy tricycles. A two-year-old can use a tricycle but will propel himself along with his feet rather than by using the pedals. He will find this great fun and by the age of three he will probably be using the pedals and be able to steer around corners. By four, your child will be able to ride his tricycle with ease and will be able to turn around sharp bends.

Teach your child at a young age to wear a helmet when riding a tricycle or other wheeled toys. As a parent or caregiver, you also should wear a helmet to model safe behavior.

Once your child has mastered riding his tricycle, he will be ready to try a bike. Some three- and four-year-old children start learning to ride a bicycle with training wheels.

Skating

Many children love to roller skate and it can help develop balancing skills. The age skating can be started depends on the individual – although many four-year-olds are able to use skates. Whatever the child's age it is important to make sure that he wears all the necessary protection – in particular a helmet as well as knee and elbow pads. Flat paths in parks are the ideal place to learn to skate.

Ball games

Even very small children love playing with balls, at first simply rolling them around,

TIME FOR A CHECK-UP

It is impossible to say for certain when children will perfect a particular skill. However, you should inform your pediatrician if by the age of five, your child cannot do the following:

- throw a ball overhand
- jump in place
- ride a tricycle

but gradually, from the age of 18 months or so, skills involving both arms and legs begin to develop. First, toddlers start to throw balls and by the time a child is two, he is likely to be able to throw a small ball overarm. As far as kicking a ball is concerned, at around two years a child will walk into a large ball but will probably not be able to kick it effectively. Over the next six months or so he will learn to give a ball a kick but it will probably travel only a short distance.

Most three-year-olds can throw a ball reasonably well overarm and can catch a large, bounced ball when their arms are held out straight. They can now kick a ball more effectively and will start to enjoy trying to kick a ball backward and forward.

By four years, children are really starting to enjoy ball games that include catching, throwing, bouncing, and kicking; they are better able to judge direction when throwing. They can catch smaller balls with their hands, and may be able to use a small bat or racquet.

By five, children play and enjoy more complex ball games.

Fitballs
A 20–26-inch exercise ball offers lots of fun-filled activities for your older child. Make certain you supervise your child at all times.

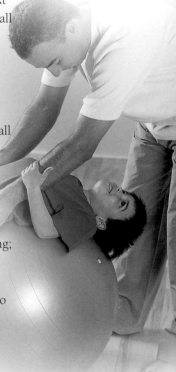

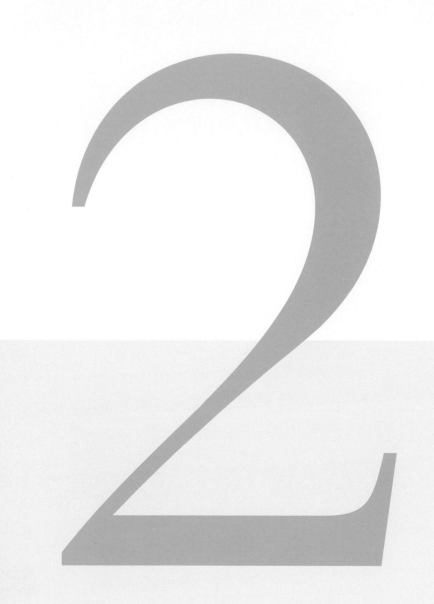
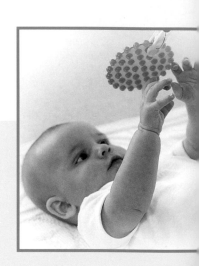

fine motor development

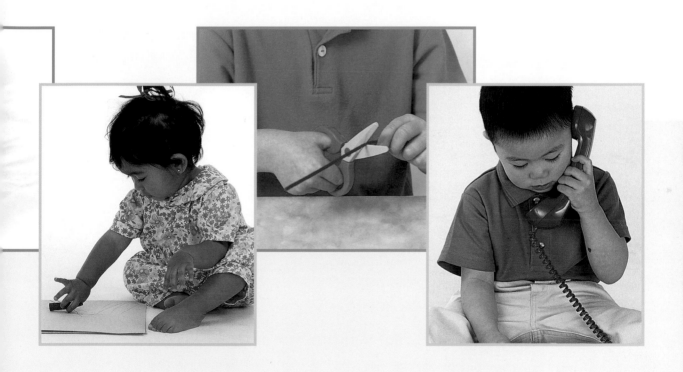

understanding the stages

The gross motor skills required for movement involve large movements of the body, arms, and legs, while the fine motor skills required for finger and hand movement involve smaller, more precise movements. The latter also depend on complex, dynamic interactions in the brain to produce the often complicated sequences needed to reach for, grab hold of, and manipulate an item. This is why fine motor control is crucial to your child's overall intellectual development.

A baby is born capable of the first stage of fine motor movement, grasping, but this is not a skill but an innate reflex, which will be lost over the next few weeks. By the age of three months, however, your baby will have learned to grasp objects deliberately and this will form the basis of the fine motor skills to follow.

What happens
Fine motor skills depend on the development of the small muscles involved in the arms and hands and the right messages being sent to them from the brain to stimulate the appropriate movements. Practicing the movements again and again strengthens the muscles as well as strengthening the nerve pathways.

Fine motor skills also rely on hand-eye coordination and spatial awareness to produce the delicate movements needed. These also improve with practice; it is only through reaching for objects many times that a baby will eventually be able to gauge the distances accurately and move her hand to just the right place.

Not only are fine motor skills an amazing achievement in their own right, they are also often performed at the same time as we move around.

The sequence of events
Fine motor control develops from the top down and from the center of the body outward – simply put, your baby will be better able to control her arm movements before those of her fingers. Due to the developments in the brain, she'll also be able to locate something using her senses of vision and hearing before she can voluntarily reach it.

Before a baby can move her hands purposefully, she must become aware that her hands are there. From around the age of two months, a baby will start to play with her hands and bring them together. From then on, she will gain further finger and hand skills rapidly, first regaining one of her newborn instincts to fold her fingers around an object and grasp it. Once your baby can grasp an object, she soon learns how to hold on to it, and then to

APPROXIMATE TIMING OF EVENTS

The key fine motor skills are acquired at approximately these ages.

2 months:	Becomes aware of own fingers.
3 months:	Holds rattle briefly when placed in hand.
4 months:	Shakes rattle to make a noise.
5 months:	Gets hold of an object using the palmar grasp. Grabs toes and pulls them to mouth.
6 months:	Reaches with one or both hands to get hold of a toy. Passes objects from one hand to the other. Brings everything to mouth.
7 months:	Starts to hold a spoon. Holds a two-handled cup and drinks from it.
8 months:	Starts to use the early pincer grip. May hold out an object but probably will not let go yet.
9 months:	Holds a string between finger and thumb and pulls toy. Takes an offered toy. Starts to let go of toys voluntarily. Points at objects, claps, and waves good-bye.
9–10 months:	Holds object in each hand and brings them together with a bang. Pincer grip becoming more refined and precise.
10 months:	Copies hair brushing.
11 months:	Lets go of objects deliberately. Enjoys passing objects back and forth.

12 months:	Refined pincer grip is used. Holds two objects in one hand. Puts objects into a container. Better at using a spoon. Picks up sippy cup and drinks from it. Throws objects but with little control or direction. Watches objects that are dropped or thrown as they fall to the ground.
15 months:	Picks up small object with either hand. Brings spoon to mouth but drops some of the food when the spoon turns over.
16–18 months:	Throws purposefully. Plays with push toys.
18 months:	Can build a three-block tower. Starts to show hand preference.
2 years:	Using preferred hand for most activities. Builds tower of six or seven blocks.
3 years:	Can handle fork. Can thread large beads. Can build tower of 9–10 blocks.
4 years:	Can use sewing cards. Can build bridges of several blocks. Will hold pencil with adult grip.
5 years:	Accomplished at drawing and painting. Can pour milk without spilling.

manipulate it by passing it from hand to hand and turning it over to examine it. She will then learn to pick objects up and later to put them down. Once the basic fine motor skills have been achieved, a child will use them in a range of creative activities, from building, drawing, and painting to looking at books and later playing musical instruments. Their developing fine motor skills also give children the ability to be independent; they gradually learn to feed and later bathe and dress themselves.

Aiding your child's progress

Babies love to touch, feel, and manipulate objects. You can encourage this from an early age by providing a variety of safe, interesting objects to play with. At first, you can help your baby explore the sensations of touch by gently opening her hands and stroking them with different fabrics, fake fur, corrugated cardboard, and feathers. Later, you can give her interesting objects to pass from hand to hand and examine. Before too long, you can let her make real use of her newfound skills by giving her finger foods to pick up and put in her mouth. You may be surprised to find how early certain activities can be introduced to your child. For example, some toddlers can start to play with crayons from about 15 months and paint from 18 months or so.

The more things she has to do with her hands, the more your child's manipulation skills will develop – and the more fun she will have.

Remember, as with all aspects of developmental learning, let your baby practice activities without feeling under any pressure. At first this will simply consist of giving her the time she needs and encouraging her both when she succeeds and when she fails. Also, sometimes let her proceed with an activity that takes her attention, knowing that you are there in the background if she needs you. As she gets older, let her lead the play sometimes; let her do what she wants with a toy rather than telling her how to play when she may have an idea of her own. For example, instead of saying "Let's build a house with these bricks," wait to see what she wants to do.

Seeking advice

The timing of milestones varies from child to child; many children will achieve the milestones before or after the "average" ages. Achieving fine motor milestones a little early may be of no consequence or may indicate that a child is going to be particularly dexterous. However, achieving these milestones a little late has probably no significance whatsoever. A more significant delay may in a few cases suggest that there is an underlying problem.

If you have any concerns, consult your pediatrician. Specifically, by around two months, your baby should be showing interest in the toys you show her. This will be encouraged by using toys in bright, contrasting colors. Mirrors and other shiny objects should also stimulate her interest. Babies should be picking toys up themselves by nine months. Remember, every child varies in their development but if either of these are not occurring by this age, you should consult your pediatrician.

reaching, grasping, and holding

Once a baby learns to grasp and hold his toys he can take a much more active role in play rather than simply watching things placed in his field of vision or swiping at toys hanging around him. At first he will hold objects but will not look at them. However, soon he will start to manipulate them, turning them over in his hands and examining them carefully. Later on, he will be able to transfer them from hand to hand. Fine motor skills are acquired rapidly in the first year and then built on in the years to come.

Grasping and holding

Grasping objects starts as a primitive reflex, but in his third month, your baby probably will start learning how to hold objects and later how to pick them up and let them go. Your baby will start to hold objects first with a palmar grasp (held in the palm of the hand between all fingers) and later with the more precise pincer grasp (held between thumb and forefinger).

For the first few weeks, your baby's hands are curled up tightly into fists most of the time. You can help relax them by massaging his palms and fingers and rubbing different-textured toys into his palms. After two months or so, his hands will begin to uncurl and he often spreads them wide. (If placed on his stomach some of the time, his arms become weight bearing which helps to extend his wrists and to open his hands.) This is when a baby starts to become aware of his hands.

Young babies (of about two to four months), deliberately grip objects pressed into their hands but may have difficulty holding small or strangely shaped items. They also find it difficult to let go of things and you may have to distract your baby with another toy to get him to let go of the first!

Get a grip
Once a baby is able to hold things, he soon accommodates his grasp to suit different-shaped objects.

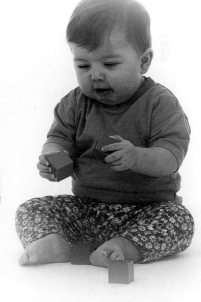

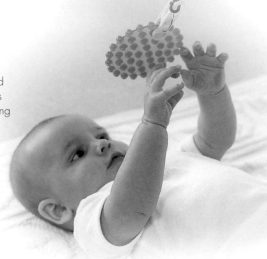

Swiping
Good eye, arm, and hand coordination is required for this young baby to manage to touch the object.

Slightly older babies will begin shaking a toy to see if it makes a sound and may be able to pass an object from one hand to another (see page 49). Soon after, babies begin to use their hands to explore the property of objects – finding out if they are hard or soft, heavy or light, and whether they make a sound.

Reaching

Before your baby's hand-eye and muscular coordination are perfected, he will reach for objects by swiping at them – usually with a clenched fist. Although he's been making lots of movements with his arms from birth, gradually you will notice that these movements become more intentional and are directed at objects that are within his reach. Though the motions seem simple enough, there's a lot of complex thinking going on! In swiping at an object, say a mobile, your baby demonstrates that he is interested in the object and what it might do. However, in order to touch the item (which he can only do using broad movements of his arm, as his hand and finger muscles develop later on), he has to formulate a plan of action and, if he elicits a response – movement and/or noise, he then has to make sense of it and see if he can repeat it or make something else happen. Later, when he can uncurl his fingers, so that he swipes with open hands, he will hit his target more often and this has the effect of spurring him on to greater efforts.

TIME FOR A CHECK-UP
If, by four to five months of age, your baby's hands remain curled into a fist and he is not able to grasp objects, you should consult your pediatrician.

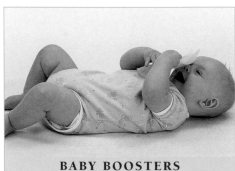

BABY BOOSTERS
ENGAGING YOUR BABY'S SENSES

Keep a stock of safe objects for your baby to hold such as books, soft blocks, wooden and plastic spoons, empty containers, plastic cups, rattles, squeeze toys, balls, or a bunch of toy keys. They may be interesting because of their texture and how they feel but also they may catch your baby's attention because they make a sound or are brightly colored.

Weeks of trial and error swiping at objects will gradually teach your baby what "works" and what doesn't and he'll become more adept at stretching out both his hands to reach for an object. However, it's not until he can sit unsupported that he'll master the further skills of accurate location (even in the dark) of an object, its size and shape for grasping, and be able to get to it even if it's moving.

You can help your baby reach for items by placing him in an infant seat and offering him toys that are in front, slightly above, or slightly below his line of sight or to the side. Encourage him to use both hands (see also page 55).

Transferring

This is an important part of learning to manipulate and play with objects. From the age of six months, babies start to pass a toy from one hand to the other and by nine months they can pass a toy frequently between the hands and turn it over so that they can examine it carefully. You can encourage this by giving your baby safe, hand-sized objects that are interesting because of their color, shape, and texture.

The stages of reaching, grasping, and holding

Holding on to objects is the natural progression from grasping them. These skills are acquired around the following ages:

* *At 2 months:* Babies of this age start to become aware of their fingers and begin to look at them when lying on their backs.

* *At 3 months:* You will probably notice your baby start to play with his fingers. He may clasp and unclasp his hands and hold

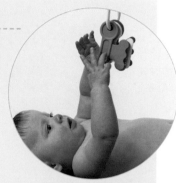
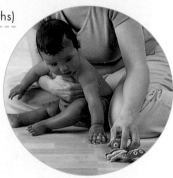

a rattle briefly when it is placed in his hand. He may also draw it toward his face but will not look at it until he is at least four months old.

✳ At 4 months: Many babies of this age can grasp a toy with two hands. Once holding a rattle they may shake it to make a noise. In this way they are starting to learn about cause and effect. Your baby may also reach out his hands to get a toy but he probably won't get hold of it right away as his hand-eye coordination is still developing.

✳ At 5 months: Babies get hold of objects in the palms of their hands (the palmar grasp). At around this age, your baby will probably grasp his toes and start to put them in his mouth.

✳ At 6 months: Babies now stretch out one or both hands to get hold of a toy. They also may be able to get hold of a cube.

✳ At 7 months: Fine motor skills are being acquired at a great rate; some babies start to hold a spoon about now.

✳ At 8 months: It is around this time that your baby may start to pick objects up with an early pincer grip, using his thumb and fingers (see page 51). The pincer grasp

That's entertainment! Lying under a mobile can be great fun for a three-month-old. He will love the variety of stimuli provided by the different colors and shapes as well as the movement he causes when he touches the toys.

EVERYTHING TO MOUTH

As soon as your baby can hold objects, he will learn to put them in his mouth. Take care to ensure that your baby doesn't get hold of anything that he could choke on or that he may push up his nose or into his ears. As well as small objects, keep larger objects out of his way if there is a chance that a small part may be pulled or chewed off. Balloons, balls less than or equal to 1¾-inch in diameter, and other similar objects can completely block a young child's throat. Most children stop putting objects in their mouths by the age of three. They may still try to push a small object into their nose or ear when they are older, so watch out!

continues to develop so that even smaller objects can be picked up between the thumb and finger. In the next year or so it will become more refined.

✳ At 9–10 months: Babies learn to hold objects in both hands at the same time and love the noise they make when they bang them together. From this time, grasping and holding are used in more and more activities, including building towers with cubes (see page 60), scribbling, and later drawing (see page 62).

✳ At around 12 months: Your baby will learn to hold two objects in one hand, so give him small (but not too small) objects to hold. At this age, babies tend to become more adept at using a spoon and will love playing with them – spoons are great for pretend feeding, banging, and later stirring.

picking up and letting go

It will be eight months or so before your baby learns to pick objects up deliberately using her thumb and fingers. Not only must she learn to pick objects up but she must also find out how to put them down instead of letting them go so that they fall to the ground.

The stages of picking up

* **Around 4 months:** Babies begin picking up objects by pressing the palms of their hands against them and curling their fingers around them.

* **At 6 months:** Hand-eye coordination is fairly well developed but your baby doesn't yet have fine motor control over her fingers. She may try to scoop up small objects by pushing them with the side of one hand onto the open palm of the other.

* **Around 8 months:** The way your baby picks objects up starts to become more refined. At this age, she will probably start to pick things up using her thumb and fingers instead of using a palmar grasp as previously. She may hold objects out toward you but will probably not know how to let go deliberately yet.

* **At 9 months:** Your baby may now reach out to take a toy from you. She is developing a pincer grasp, by which she picks up objects between her thumb and first finger.

* **At 12 months:** One-year-olds can pick small objects up skillfully with a pincer grasp using their thumbs and first fingers. This is a key milestone and will enable

them to pick up objects more easily. Later, similar positions of the hand will be used when writing, drawing, and painting as well as buttoning and zipping clothes.

* **At 15 months:** By now most toddlers can pick up a small object with great accuracy using either hand.

* **From 2–4 years:** During this period, dexterity improves greatly and is helped along as children develop many new fine motor skills. They learn to pick up and put down objects carefully and by age four are happy picking up tiny objects.

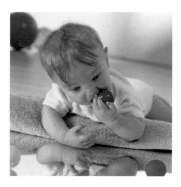

The developing grasp
Up to six months of age, your baby will hold a ball in the palm of his hand; at eight months he'll hold it between fingers and thumb, and eventually between thumb and forefinger only.

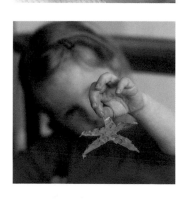

Pick and choose

By 12 months, your baby will probably be able to put objects in a container. Try giving her a basket or large cardboard box with a selection of objects to put in and take out. From around this age, she can start to help you to unpack your shopping bag. She will also love playing with an old handbag full of interesting objects.

Toy toss
Babies always seem to delight in throwing their toys. By doing so, they are learning a lot about how things work. It may make a noise, it may bounce, but it won't come back by itself!

Dropping and putting down

From the time (about four months of age) when a baby starts to learn to hold objects, she also will drop them. At this stage and for some months to come, out of sight out of mind will be the state of affairs – once something is dropped it will be forgotten. It will not be until the age of about a year that your baby will watch the toys that she drops and throws fall to the ground. She also will begin to look in the right place for objects that have fallen out of sight (see also page 78).

From about nine months, your baby may start to let go of objects voluntarily. At first she will drop them, but over the next three months or so, she will learn to press them against a tabletop or other surface before releasing them, and also to throw objects when she has had enough of them. It will be some months before she will learn to put objects down carefully using a pincer grasp.

Throwing

This is another way of getting rid of unwanted objects. Most year-old babies are able to throw objects but it's not until they are 18 months old that babies start to throw with some purpose. In fact, it may be one of your baby's favorite activities to throw things and call for you to retrieve them. At this age, you can try giving your toddler a ball to throw. Whether she is crawling or walking, she also will enjoy going to retrieve the ball.

EXTRA CAUTIOUS
Take extra precautions now that your baby can pick things up using a pincer grasp. Pills, beads, coins, and other small items can be dangerous and potentially life threatening to an infant or toddler. Cover all electrical sockets to prevent her from poking fingers or objects inside.

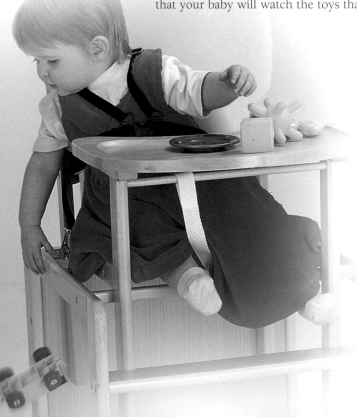

other hand and finger skills

There will be a number of other useful skills your baby will pick up along the way. As with the basic manipulation skills, you can provide the opportunity for him to practice through play.

Pulling and pushing

Once your baby can keep hold of something, he will, within a few months, learn to pull it along. At nine months, many babies can get hold of a string between their fingers and thumbs to pull a toy toward them. Over the next few months they will learn to pull toys along. By a year or so, they will start to love playing with pull toys. These will be a particular favorite between the ages of one and two years.

Toddlers will usually start to play with push toys between the ages of 15 and 18 months. These can be great to give some support to the early walker. Push toys must be stable and strong enough to support a toddler in his early walking.

Pointing

By the age of nine months, babies have started to move their fingers individually. This is a great achievement, which will enable them to pick objects up using their thumbs and fingers as well as pointing at objects and people. Pointing is one of the ways your baby communicates (see also page 101). At nine months, he will start to point toward things in the distance that he'll want you to get for him. By the age of one year, he'll be using his index finger to point out things to you that he finds interesting. You can encourage this behavior by starting to point out things of interest such as cars and animals. Babies will love to hear the names of the animals and the noises they make. Your baby will start to copy pointing and eventually will make attempts at naming them. In this way you are encouraging your baby to develop a fine motor skill while using his visual skills and paving the way for the introduction of words in the future.

Clapping and waving

Babies learn to clap hands at around the age of nine months. They also learn to wave

Look at me!
This baby is able to use her hands and fingers to point, clap, and wave, but if she waves too hard she may fall over as she's not quite mastered upright sitting.

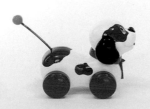

good-bye at about this age. Play music and sing songs while clapping along to the rhythm to encourage your baby to join in. Babies love to copy, so find songs that have actions, including waving bye-bye.

Turning and unscrewing

By 18 months, many toddlers are able to turn the pages of a book, if only a few at a time. By age two, children enjoy looking at more detailed books and can turn pages individually. Looking at books and encouraging your child to enjoy them will prepare him for the time he learns to read.

Around the age of two, children learn about turning knobs and will enjoy toys that incorporate knobs. Learning this turning movement also means they are able to unscrew lids.

Unwrapping

Between the ages of two and two and a half years children learn to unwrap objects. From this age your child will love to wrap up objects with you as pretend presents for dolls and stuffed animals and

Copying

Babies mimic what we do and that's the way they learn many of their skills. By 12 months many will know the actions needed to use a telephone. As well as helping to improve dexterity, toy phones also encourage children in early speech as they soon copy the sounds you make when using the telephone.

CHILD LOCKS

Before your baby is able to unscrew and turn things, you must fully childproof your home. If you haven't already done this, do it now. Special child locks are available for cupboards, drawers, and doors. Even with these, it is important to ensure you store everything breakable or potentially dangerous well out of your child's reach.

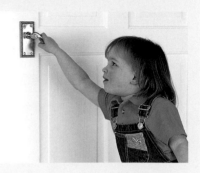

then open them up again. When your child is older (three to four years) you can make a pretend gift for a doll's birthday party and have fun playing together.

PARENTAL PARTICIPATION

Ring-around-the-rosy

From around the age of two years, toddlers will be able to perform games and songs that require action. However, babies as young as six months will enjoy them too, even if they are unable to copy all the actions. From the age of one or so, babies will love to clap when listening to music.

handedness

Although handedness isn't completely clear-cut until about three years of age, toddlers usually start to show a preference for using either their right or left hands at about 18 months, and by two years they tend to use their preferred hand for most activities. A one-year-old usually uses both hands equally.

More than 90 percent of people are right-handed. A small number of people can use either hand for all activities (known as being ambidextrous) whereas some use one hand for certain activities and the other hand for others. A child who has a left-handed parent has an increased likelihood of being left-handed but she is still more likely to be right-handed. If both parents are left-handed the chance of the child being left-handed is increased further.

What determines handedness?

It has not yet been established whether it is genes that determine handedness or whether it is due to as-yet-unidentified factors, such as asymmetry in the brain. It is interesting to note that identical twins do not necessarily have the same hand preference. This supports the theory that handedness is not a matter of simple genetic inheritance.

One recent study suggested that handedness may develop in the uterus during pregnancy rather than in the first years of childhood as was previously thought. Fetal ultrasound scans were examined; 90 percent of those of 15 weeks gestation were seen to suck their right thumbs, the others sucked their left. A number of the fetuses were observed for

years after birth and at age 10 or older, all of those who had sucked their right thumbs went on to be right-handed and two-thirds of those who had sucked their left thumbs went on to be left-handed, the others being right-handed.

The question remains unanswered as to why the preference for one hand seems to take three to four years to be fully established if it is present so early in life.

Should anything be done?

Handedness develops naturally and there is nothing a parent should do to help this along. What you can do, once a preference for the left hand is shown, is to provide special equipment, such as left-handed scissors, for your child. Otherwise those who are left-handed have no special requirements. Handedness has no influence on the ability to learn.

TIME FOR A CHECK-UP
If your baby shows a preference for using one hand more than the other before the age of 12 months, let your pediatrician know. There may in a few cases be an underlying problem.

coordinating objects

Another fine motor milestone is when your baby learns to control (or manipulate) more than one object at a time. This occurs when he hits two blocks together, for example. Soon he will "graduate" to fitting things together – and taking them apart, threading objects, and trying more dexterous activities.

Initially, your baby will use one object, such as a spoon, to hit another, which is fixed and unmoving, such as his feeding tray, but soon he will be able to bring two objects together, one in each hand. The latter is a difficult task as it involves simultaneously coordinating the movements in both of his arms and hands. Your baby is usually only capable of doing this once he can sit up confidently unsupported.

Once your baby has learned about impact, he will try experimenting with threading objects, fitting things together, and finally building.

Making music
Ordinary household objects can be used to shake, rattle, and bang.

Banging
Hitting one object against another not only produces noise but allows your baby to make lots of interesting discoveries about how things work.

From the age of two or so, toddlers can bang on a drum with two sticks. They may also be able to make music with a simple xylophone. Try a wooden xylophone, which makes a more mellow sound, much easier on the ear than the plastic and metal instruments.

Two-year-olds also love to play with toy hammers, perhaps banging balls through holes. Babies as young as 12 months can give this sort of activity a try but make sure the hammer is a light, plastic one. One-year-olds have a strong grip and so can use a hammer to bash pegs into a peg table.

Putting things together
From around 18 months toddlers will try to put the pieces of a simple toy together. You will be able to do two- or three-piece jigsaw puzzles together. Fitting objects one inside the other or piling them up and pushing them down also are fascinating activities for 18-month-olds. Other toys are available that encourage simple construction, such as a railway track made

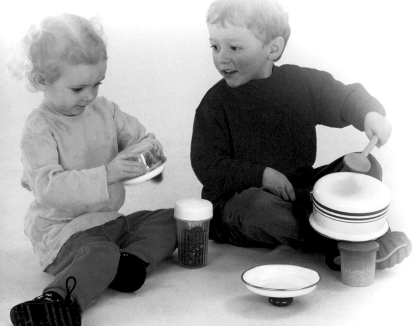

up of large pieces that easily fit together. Around this age, many toddlers will really start to enjoy playing with cars and trains. You can draw a simple road or track on a large piece of paper or wallpaper for them to follow. Draw on houses, shops, and a garage to make the play more interesting or place toy buildings on the paper for the cars to navigate around.

Threading and sewing

Threading is a great pastime for young children and can be started around the age of two, when some children can thread spools or tubes onto a piece of string or yarn.

Many three year olds can thread large beads onto a shoelace and by four, your child may be able to place big buttons onto

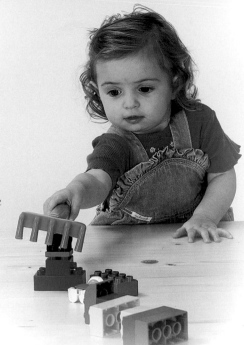

"Tool" use Clever planning and understanding is demonstrated when your toddler employs objects to achieve a goal, such as using one toy to reach another farther away or to push away food she doesn't like.

a thread with a blunt plastic needle. Sewing can begin from the age of four or so and sewing cards are a simple and fun way to learn. You can buy them or make your own by drawing a shape on a piece of card and cutting holes in the outline, perhaps with a hole punch. Always use a blunt plastic needle and thread it with yarn to sew around the outline.

Cooking

You will probably find your child loves helping you with the cooking from about the age of three. There are plenty of things he can do to exercise his newfound dexterity. He can help assemble salad ingredients, will love mixing, and should be able to roll out dough and use simple cookie cutters with it. He will be able to help you decorate cakes and cookies with icing pens.

encouraging the artist in your child

Children can start to enjoy being creative from quite an early age. Many can use crayons from about 15 months and will love playing with paints from about 18 months. Two year olds love finger painting and making prints with their hands and feet, while three year olds love sponge painting and potato printing.

Craft activities will help your child develop her fine motor skills, particularly those of cutting and molding. Using color and texture and exploring a wide variety of materials will help develop her aesthetic appreciation and artistic abilities. Most importantly, creating art will enable you and your child to spend many exciting and interesting hours together.

Age-appropriate activities

Three-year-olds will enjoy working with clay and play dough, although what she makes may not be easily recognizable. Encourage her to use her painting and printing skills to make greeting cards and other "gift items." She'll be pleased if you display her work. Four-year-olds will enjoy cutting paper with child safety scissors and can make simple collages. They also like dressing up, so making appropriate props for costumes will be appreciated.

Five-year-olds can copy designs and shapes and will be ready for more detailed arts and crafts including simple model making using papier mâché. Supervise art activities and provide only safe art materials.

Craft materials

Have on hand a selection of plain and differently colored paper of various thicknesses, glue, crayons, and paints. Decorate this with beads, ribbon, pipe cleaners, sequins, glitter, dried peas and beans, and plastic packing materials. Items previously collected, such as feathers, pine cones, seed cases, leaves, and shells, also may come in handy.

Play dough
Although an 18-month-old toddler will enjoy

MAKING PLAY DOUGH

- 2 cups plain flour
- 1 cup salt
- 1 cup water
- 2 tbs. olive oil
- 2 tsps. cream of tartar (this makes the dough last longer)

Mix these together and warm them in a pan on the stove. Let the mixture cool down a little and then form it into a ball before kneading it for a few minutes. Remember to soak the pan immediately before the remnants become caked on. Food coloring can be added.

The dough will last for a few months as long as it is kept in a plastic bag or an airtight plastic box to prevent it from drying out.

making simple shapes from play dough, it won't be until your child is about three that she'll be able to use simple toys to cut and shape it. "Pretend cooking" is a favorite activity; your child can roll out the dough and use cookie cutters to make pretend cookies. She also can use it to make models – if you want to keep them they need to be baked in a medium oven until they are hard (this usually takes about 15 minutes). Once they are cold, they can be decorated with poster paints.

Seasonal fun
Many activities can help your child celebrate the seasons. For older children, a blown-up balloon covered in torn newspaper strips applied with glue can be painted to form a colorful jack-o'-lantern for Halloween fun.

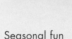

MINIMIZING MESS

Making a mess is part of the fun of being creative when you are a child. Try not to worry too much as this time together should be fun. Clothes can easily be protected by wearing an old shirt of yours worn backward or an apron. A low table is great to work on and can be covered with old newspaper or a plastic cloth. It is also worth covering the floor underneath with plastic sheeting.

For young children, go for thick paints poured into a paint pot or other container. You can buy paint pots in stands that will not topple over.

building

As with the more basic manipulation skills, building is acquired in a series of stages beginning at the age of around 18 months, when toddlers learn to build a three-block tower. However, it can start earlier as some 12-month-old children can put one block on top of another to make a small tower.

When you see your child attempting to build a tower, you should bear in mind that this is a considerable achievement. He is demonstrating that he knows what he wants to do, he's probably copied your example, and he has the necessary skills to carry it out. Encourage your child's building skills; they are a great way to improve dexterity and control as well as developing spatial awareness and visual skills. Building also shows your child's willingness to practice an activity again and again as he will try to build a tower many times despite the fact it will repeatedly fall over. However, block use is not limited to building. Other skills that development specialists deem important are the construction of play steps, bridges, and objects such as trains and houses.

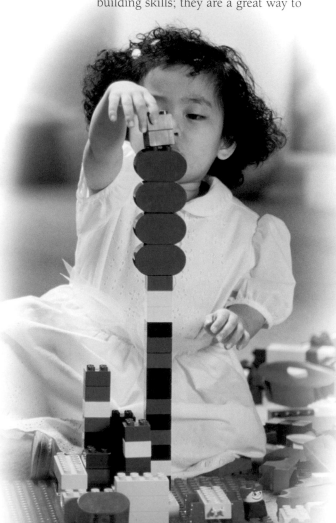

Building with blocks

Although toddlers start building small towers at around 18 months, they will enjoy playing with soft blocks from an earlier age. Soft blocks can be used for squeezing, throwing, and building.

* *Around 9 months:* Babies are able to hold a small block in both hands and find banging them together very satisfying.
* *Around 18 months:* Your toddler may build a three-block tower, but will need to follow an example. Within a few weeks, he will be happy to do this all by himself.
* *Around 2 years:* Many toddlers can build a tower of six or seven blocks, again first following a demonstration.
* *By the age of 2½:* Your toddler will probably be able to build a tower of seven or more cubes using his preferred hand.

* By 3 years: This will increase to nine or 10 cubes and

* By 4 years: 10 or more. Throughout this time, however, a great deal of fun will be gained from knocking the tower to the ground before starting again.

As well as towers, small children enjoy building bridges. They start with bridges of three cubes with or without a demonstration. They also learn to build three steps with six cubes. By the age of three or four, children can build a bridge of three bricks with either hand and by four years, they can build higher steps and other more complex models with blocks.

Building toys

Various toys are available that allow babies and young toddlers to practice stacking before they acquire the necessary skills for true building.

Nesting containers are a particular favorite with one-year-olds. As well as enabling them to practice their building skills, they also allow them to use another skill developed at around this age – putting one object inside another. These make great containers for putting other objects in, cups for "let's pretend" (add a plastic pitcher for a simple tea set), and for pouring water in the bath.

Young toddlers also enjoy placing rings on spindle toys (with or without a rocking base) or over boards with wooden rods of different heights. As well as developing their hand and finger manipulation skills, these simple toys give your child practice with shape discrimination.

As with all toys for this age group, look for containers or stacking toys of contrasting bright colors.

Around 18 months, toddlers also can start to put large linking blocks (such as Duplo™) together. This is something you can enjoy with your toddler. Encourage him to make towers and incorporate small plastic figures and animals into your play – you could help your child to make a house or stable for them. This is early "let's pretend" and playing in this way will continue to be a great pastime as your child gets older and "graduates" to other linking blocks (such as LEGO™) when his pretend play becomes more sophisticated.

From four, your child will enjoy other types of construction toys, including those with smaller and more realistic pieces, such as cars and planes he can assemble himself. Make sure, however, that these are age-appropriate for your child and that he plays with smaller pieces under supervision.

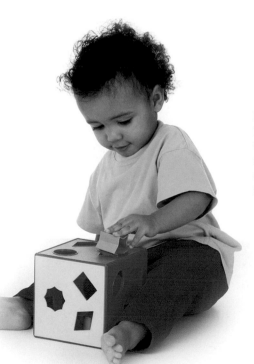

Nesting toys
These have the advantage of being able to stack up as well as fitting one within the other.

Learning aids
Blocks are not only fun to play with but can teach a child a great deal about shape, texture, and color.

drawing and cutting

Children love to be creative and this starts when a toddler first grasps hold of a crayon and then starts to scribble. Gradually, your child's drawings will become more sophisticated as she begins to create more recognizable figures, and eventually, as her pictures become more meaningful, she will start writing.

The stages of drawing

Your baby may grasp a crayon as early as 15 months. At this stage she will use the palmar grasp, holding the crayon against her palm with her fingers curled around it. For the first six months or more, her artwork will consist of scribbles backward and forward on the page. This is a recognized developmental stage; health professionals often will ask parents what their child draws at a given age as part of their assessment.

Gradually, your child's grip on the crayon or pencil will change.

* *At around 18 months:* She may hold a pencil either around the middle or near the upper end. She may use her whole hand or hold the pencil between her thumb and fingers. She will continue to scribble back and forth but also may make dots on the paper. Your toddler may hold her pencil in either hand or in both hands.

* *At 2 years:* Most children scribble around and around in circles as well as back and forth. They may be able to copy a vertical line and possibly a V shape.

Most two-year-olds hold their pencils toward the point between their thumb and first two fingers. Others may continue to hold their pencils like a dagger and even some older children do this. Two-year-olds may use a preferred hand for most of the time although it will be some time before handedness is definitely established (see page 55).

BABY BOOSTERS
COLORING CHOICE

You can start to give your child paper and crayons from the age of 15–18 months. Choose chubby crayons, which are particularly easy for little hands to hold; make sure they are nontoxic wax crayons. Give small children only a few colors at a time; they are only drawing simply at this stage and one or two colors will be sufficient.

* **At 2½ years:** Your child will probably hold her pencil in her preferred hand. She will probably copy a circle and a horizontal as well as a vertical line.

* **At 3 years:** Your child will hold her pencil near the point; the positioning of her hand will be more similar to the adult grip now with a pencil being held between her thumb and first two fingers. In addition to drawing circles, your child also may be able to copy a cross. She may draw a figure with a head and two other parts. She will not be able to plan what she is going to draw or to tell you what she will draw before she starts but is more likely to tell you what she has drawn after she has finished.

She will paint with a large brush and cut with child safety scissors.

* **At 4 years:** Your child will use the adult grip to hold her pencil. She can draw a person with a head, body, legs, and often arms and even fingers. She also can draw a simple house. She will probably be able to tell you what she is going to draw before she draws it.

* **At 5 years:** She will be accomplished at drawing and painting. She uses a pen well and probably will be able to write as well as draw. She will love painting and be able to paint skillfully with fine brushes. She can copy many letters and a square. She may be able to write letters herself without copying an example.

She will draw a person and give him facial features. She will also draw a house with a door, windows, roof, and chimney. She will draw many other things and know what she is going to draw. She will color neatly, keeping the color within the outline. In the next few months she will learn to copy a triangle.

Writing

About the time your child begins to create meaningful pictures – two and a half -– she'll start pretend "writing." Instead of the many different types of sweeping hand movements she usually makes, she'll begin to lift her pencil off the paper at regular intervals in order to create a series of small marks, some of which may be in a line.

Painting partners
Most children enjoy coloring in tandem with their parents. Although your toddler will love playing with paints from about 18 months, she will not be able to control a paintbrush and may be better using paint pens at this early age.

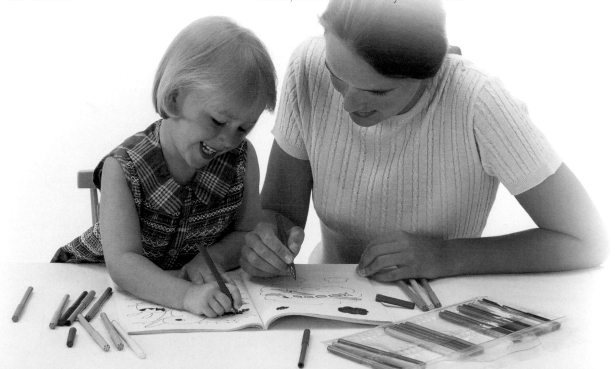

She may be able to copy a V shape and a T. She'll have watched your hand actions when you write and begun to imitate them. By age four, she can copy several letters – T, H, V, O – and at age five will be able to copy C, Y, U, among others, and write a few letters spontaneously.

This is a good time to teach her to write her name.

Cutting

Children can start to cut with blunt-ended child safety scissors when they are over two years old. This is a complex skill that takes time to acquire – a child must move the scissors forward and open and close them while directing them to the right place. Children are usually able to cut reasonably accurately by about the age of three years.

At first, you can make cutting easy by giving your child pieces of colored paper to cut into small pieces. These can be glued to a piece of paper to make a picture. By three, children can cut out a simple outline.

Craft skills
By four, children become more effective at using scissors. This makes it possible for them to engage in a lot of artistic activities such as collage making.

Sticky fun

Glueing is great fun for young kids – they can usually do it from the age of two or so. Collect fun items to stick on paper, such as pieces of shiny paper, feathers, and tissue paper.

If your child is very young, cover a piece of paper with child craft glue and show her that if she drops things onto the paper they stick. You can use flour and water glue for this. Later, your child will learn to apply the glue to the back of things and stick them on deliberately – she can use a glue stick for this.

Drawing fun

Children love to draw around their hands and feet. Supply your child with paper and pencil and show her how to trace around her feet and hands. Your child will be able to do it well from around three but will enjoy trying earlier. Encourage her to color the outlines in or fill them by sticking on small pieces of colored paper.

Three-year-olds also can use stencils. Try making your own simple stencils by cutting shapes out of a card.

self-feeding and dressing

Even before your child has developed sufficient manual dexterity to effectively feed and dress himself, he will begin to take control of these areas of his life. What comes easily to adults is much more difficult for a toddler. Essentially, for everything he does, he needs to work out a plan of action and then try to achieve it even though many movements are still unperfected.

Eating

From the time your baby starts on solids, you can encourage him to feed himself. At around eight months or so, you can offer your baby some simple finger foods, such as chunks of ripe banana, crackers, or small pieces of chicken. Although your baby may not actually be able to get much of them into his mouth, he will enjoy handling the food.

At 9 months: When you are feeding your baby, he may start to try to get hold of the spoon. This can become frustrating for you as mealtimes can easily become a battle over the spoon. It is, therefore, worth having two spoons – one for your baby to play with and one for you to feed him with. As he refines his pincer grasp (see page 51), your baby will enjoy picking up smaller and firmer pieces of food such as cooked pasta pieces, O-shaped cereal, or small rice cakes, with his fingers.

Between 11 and 14 months: Your child will want to use his own spoon to feed himself. Because he grasps the spoon as he would a toy – with a viselike grip, he won't be able to angle it properly to his mouth and instead may use it to bang on the feeding table or plate. A lot of the time, he'll just use his fingers. He's capable of picking up very small morsels of food using his thumb and forefinger.

From around 15 months: He'll start to be able to bring food to his mouth with the spoon but often the spoon will turn over at the crucial moment so that quite a bit of food won't make it into his mouth. He also may decide that using the spoon to fling food around the room is more fun.

Around 18 months: Your baby will have learned to tilt his wrist and adjust his grip, so he'll be better able to control his spoon. He holds his spoon horizontally, raising his elbow as he lifts the spoon to his mouth. He often uses his free hand to help push food into his mouth or to put spilled food on his spoon. Loading his spoon with food remains difficult as it involves coordinating several movements – reaching, grasping, and scooping – with opening his mouth at the right time. It's no wonder that meal times become messy! As you clean up yet again, try to bear in mind that this is an

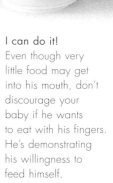

I can do it!
Even though very little food may get into his mouth, don't discourage your baby if he wants to eat with his fingers. He's demonstrating his willingness to feed himself.

important part of learning new skills and gaining more independence.

* **By 3 years:** Your toddler should be able to handle a fork and spoon with some dexterity but will need help with a knife, particularly in cutting up large pieces of food. Some toddlers may be slower at holding a spoon adult fashion, with their palms turned inward; they are more likely to keep their palms downward and lift their elbows.

* **At 4 years:** Your child will be able to eat skillfully with a knife and fork.

Drinking

The age at which your child may begin drinking from a cup can depend as much on emotional issues as his fine motor development. If he finds feeding from the breast or bottle extremely pleasurable, he may be reluctant to drink from a cup, even though he has acquired the skills.

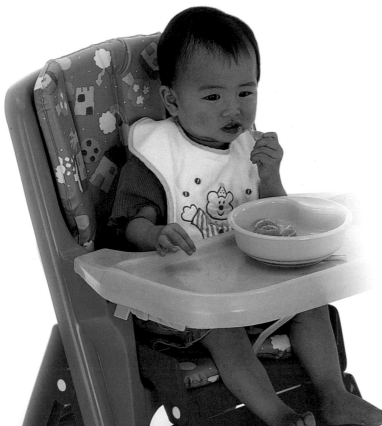

Introducing the high chair
Many babies can use a highchair from six months or so, when they are able to sit well supported in the chair. Sitting in a high chair offers your baby a safe way to practice picking up food to feed herself.

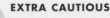
EXTRA CAUTIOUS

Infants and children can easily choke on food, especially when self-feeding. Be certain to supervise meal and snack time and insist that your infant or child eat while sitting down. Do not give your child younger than four years of age any round, firm food unless it is chopped completely. Learn CPR and talk to your pediatrician about preventing choking and what to do if it should occur.

* **From 7 months:** Your baby may drink from a cup but you will have to hand him the cup and hold it while he does so.

* **Around 9 months:** He will put his hands around a cup or bottle when feeding.

* **Around 12 months:** He will be able to pick up and hold his trainer cup himself. He won't, however, be able to put his cup down until he's older and, if you are not there to take it from him, he will drop it onto the floor.

* **Around 18 months:** He will drink from his cup, using both hands, and put it down without much spilling.

* **Around 2 years:** He will be able to hold a small glass with both his hands.

* **Around 3 years:** Your child will hold a cup by its handle and will no longer need his other hand to help.

* **Around 4½ years:** Your child can pour milk from a pitcher without spilling.

Putting on clothes

As young as 18 months, your child may start to help as you get him dressed, at first by reaching out his arms to go into sleeves.

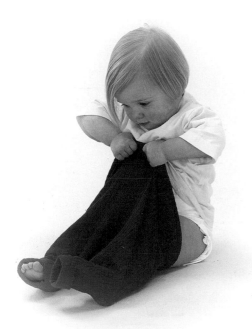

He also may try to undress himself and may be able to do this with some help from around the age of two.

Many two-year-olds are adept at removing hats, mittens, and socks.

Three year olds continue to be better at undressing than dressing but your child should be able to put on his pants, socks, and shoes. Often, however, he may put on a shirt backward and will have trouble with buttons.

By around four years, your child will be able to put on most of his clothes on his own, though it's a good idea to lay out his clothes to help him put them on correctly. However, help may be needed with tricky zippers (though some two-year-olds may be able to do them), buttons, and shoelaces. Some four-year-olds can even do and undo their own buckles.

PARENTAL PARTICIPATION

Many three- and four-year-olds turn getting dressed into a battle. You can defuse a potentially difficult situation or build confidence in your child by doing the following.

Give him a choice

If your child dislikes certain clothes or tends to choose inappropriate items (shorts in midwinter), let him choose between two items. "Would you rather wear these pants or jeans today?" This makes him feel he is part of the decision as well as distracting him from the item that is best forgotten.

Provide practice

Young children love to do new things and this includes learning how to work zippers, buttons, and buckles. Look for items around the house that will allow your child to practice, such as a make-up bag with a zipper. Cards are available that teach children to lace up and later to tie simple knots and bows.

Dressing-up box

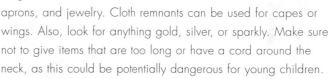

From around the age of three or even earlier, children love to dress up. Young children will get a lot of pleasure from wearing your old clothes and accessories around the house. Collect everything you have in a large box – the greater the variety the better. Look for old scarves, gloves, hats, sunglasses, old dresses, shoes, feather boas, aprons, and jewelry. Cloth remnants can be used for capes or wings. Also, look for anything gold, silver, or sparkly. Make sure not to give items that are too long or have a cord around the neck, as this could be potentially dangerous for young children.

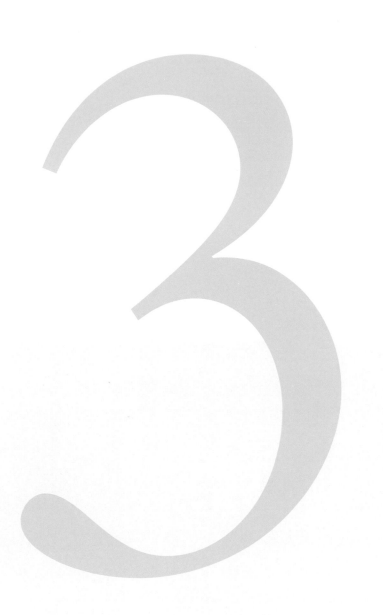

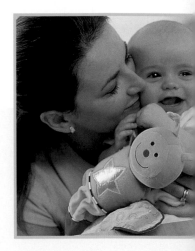

sensory
development

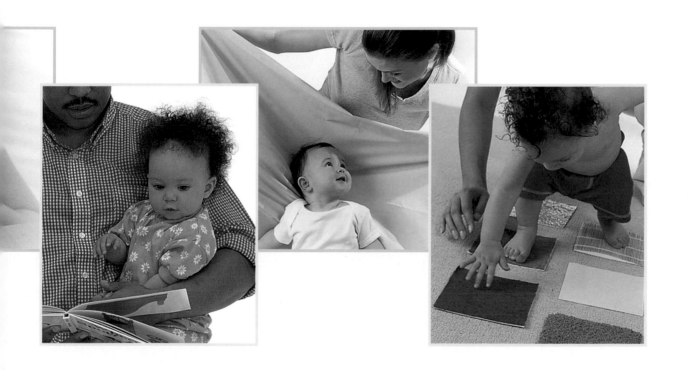

understanding the stages

Throughout childhood, your growing infant uses her sensory skills to process information, learn new concepts, organize and understand experiences, and derive pleasure from her environment. Although these senses are well developed by the age of five, most of the elementary sensory skills were already established to some extent when she arrived in the world. These basic senses are sight, hearing, smelling, tasting, touch, and motion sensitivity.

Keep it fun
Stimulation during childhood is a serious business but your baby takes in much more through his senses when he enjoys himself. Be relaxed when you play, and laugh in response to his delighted squeals.

Your child's ever-increasing perceptual skills, which steadily develop from birth onward, are only possible because of the rapid growth of her brain and central nervous system. At birth, your baby's brain size was roughly 25 percent of its eventual full adult weight, but by the age of two, it has increased to 75 percent of its full adult weight. That's quite a surge in brain capacity in the space of only a couple of years. However, it's not just brain development that takes place. There is also growth in the spinal cord and the nerves, which supports her perceptual system.

That part of the brain that controls the basic senses grows quickest during the first year, which is why perceptual skills extend so rapidly during this period.

Your baby's basic senses are active from the very moment she arrives. She has been biologically preprogrammed to respond to her environment using all her five senses. When she is born, she is sensitive to:

* *Light.* If a very bright light shines into her eyes, she shuts them tightly and keeps them that way until the light is removed.

* *Sound.* She reacts more to a human voice than to any other sound. She tells the difference between a real cry and a machine-made sound.
* *Touch.* Your baby turns her mouth toward your fingertip, when you gently stroke the side of her cheek with it.
* *Smell.* She very quickly learns the difference between the smell of her mother's breast milk and the smell of someone else's breast milk.
* *Taste.* She may spit out her milk if it's not at exactly the right temperature, or if it tastes different from her usual feeding.

Sensory combination

Each of the senses grows individually and has its own characteristics, but your growing child typically combines at least two or more senses every time she interacts or explores. For instance, when your infant plays with a rattle, she holds it (touch), shakes it (motion), looks at it (sight), listens to its noise (hearing), and may even bite it (taste) or sniff it (smell). Information from these different senses blend to give her an overall concept of the object in front of her, using two separate higher-order perceptual skills.

Sensory integration is your child's ability to integrate different information from different senses at the same time; for example, she watches you speak to her and is able to match your voice sounds with your lip movements.

Cross-modal transfer is your baby's ability to learn something through one sense and then transfer it to another, for instance, she feels a toy without seeing it, and then is able to identify that toy by sight alone.

Both these perceptual skills are present in a newborn to some extent, and they become consolidated and mature over the following five years.

Perceptual learning

As your child progresses through the different stages of perceptual development, it's not simply that her individual sensory skills improve, it's also that she learns from her perceptual experiences. In other words, she begins to gather knowledge from using her different senses; she builds new understanding from them.

For instance, at first, your two-year-old probably can't tell the difference between, say, two dogs that are the same color and height. As far as she is concerned, they are both the same. Through experience, perhaps by touching them, stroking them, looking at them, listening to their barks, or even smelling them, she gradually learns their distinctive features and is able to tell them apart.

Your child actively uses information gained from the senses to learn about her

- -

In the know... Bonding aids

Each of her senses individually enables your baby to start learning from day one. But together they enable her to form an emotional attachment to you and your partner, which is crucial to her overall development. By interacting with you through sight, sound, hearing, smell, and taste, your baby forms a connection with you, and this makes her feel safe and secure. Also known as "bonding," this process lays the foundation for your baby's future social and emotional development. The significance of this attachment – which is only made possible because of your newborn's use of the five senses – cannot be overestimated.

- -

world. As she progresses through the pre-school years, this form of perceptual learning becomes stronger and her ability to differentiate between a broad range of different sights, sounds, taste, smells, and touches constantly improves.

Whole-part perception

One of the sensory characteristics that separates, say, a five-year-old child from a two-year-old toddler is the ability to focus on a specific feature rather than the whole object. For instance, a younger child might say that an orange and a ball of string are the same because their overall image is roughly the same. However, an older child is less likely to group these two items together, because she looks at the specific features of each item and immediately sees that one is food and one is not, that one is white and one is orange.

Another general change in perceptual development that occurs during the early years is the way children recognize faces. Psychologists have demonstrated that younger children recognize a face using

Individual differences in rates of development are perfectly normal and, therefore, the following milestones should be regarded as guidelines not absolute points. However, if your child seems significantly delayed in achieving any of these milestones, make an appointment with your child's pediatrician.

At birth:
Sensitive to loud noises; soothed by sounds with low tones.
Notices the differences between light and dark; looks at where white and black join.
Feels pain when skin is pricked by a needle.
Has more taste buds than an adult.
Reacts negatively to foul smells.

2 months:
Watches a toy that moves slowly across line of vision.
Social smiling (smiles in response to another's).

3 months:
Distinguishes between different colors, such as red and blue.
Starts to get excited when favorite song or music is heard.
Tells the difference between taste of regular feeding and a new feed.
Shows distinct preferences for particular smells.

6 months:
Smiles when shown a photograph of herself.
Looks for longer periods of time at objects which attract her attention.
Knows the difference between the male and female voice.
Listens closely when she hears her own name mentioned.
Likes an increased range of tastes, as solids are introduced.
Can be soothed by loving, gentle touch.

9 months:
Responds to own name.
Plays peekaboo.
Searches for hidden objects.

1 year:
Concentrates better when listening to favorite story.
Listens and points to a familiar item when named.
Responds to simple one-step commands.
Pours water from a cup into basin.
Returns affectionate hugs with own cuddles.

2 years:
Studies closely pictures in books.
Recognizes own image in a photograph.
Opens boxes in order to discover what is inside.
Listens attentively to other people's conversations.
Does own form of dance to familiar music.
Can develop fussy eating habits.

3 years:	Knows the difference between a large object and a small object.
	Turns pages and closely watches them while doing so.
	Sorts objects according to shape.
	Matches items of the same color.
	Listens and responds to questions.
	Enthusiastic when a story is read.
4 years:	Names a few colors accurately.
	Enjoys the sounds of words that rhyme with each other.
	Remembers parts of a story.
	Concentrates quietly when completing a small puzzle.
	More willing to eat food if helps prepare it.
5 years:	Takes part appropriately in conversations.
	Listens closely to unfamiliar sounds and noises.
	When asked, will give name and address.
	Concentrates so hard that may ignore instructions to stop.
	Uses physical comfort to calm a crying friend.
	Has established definite food preferences.

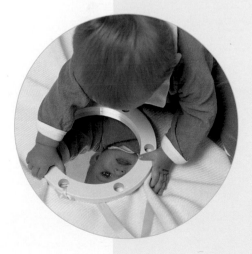

Mirror fun
Babies aged four to seven months find mirrors sources of endless fascination and sensory information.

outer cues, such as hair, chin, and head shape, while older children pay more attention to inner facial cues such as eyes, nose, and mouth.

Aiding your child's progress

Although your child has a built-in growth program that naturally drives her development, stimulation plays a huge part, too, so what you do with your child counts. That's why you need to talk to her, play with her, and let her explore. Make sure, however, that you keep play activities fun. If she senses that you are tense and anxious because she can't complete a task, she'll give up trying. Your confidence will boost her self-confidence. Always avoid confrontation. If your child resists an activity, leave it and return to it later.

Bear in mind, though, that your child doesn't need an intensive, planned program of sensory stimulation. Everything in her typical daily routine is exciting and interesting for her. Every sensory experience advances her perceptual skills one way or another.

Your child is a unique person, with her own blend of personality, abilities, and characteristics. That not only makes her special but also determines how she will develop. It's very important, therefore, to avoid comparing your child with others. Your child's development will have times of rapid pace and times of slow pace. There is no need to worry if she stays at the same point for a few weeks. You should look for all-around progress instead of concentrating on one aspect of her progress only. What matters is that you are satisfied your growing child is generally developing well.

visual skills

Your child's vision consists of a number of skills, all of which are present to some extent in your baby during his first year. However, as he gets older, the way your child uses his visual skills will change.

How your baby sees

Your baby is able to see right from birth because his eyes are designed to allow him to focus on objects and faces. His eyes are capable of the following skills:

* *Pupil change.* This is a natural reflex designed to protect his vision. When a bright light shines in his eyes, his pupil automatically slowly grows smaller and when it is dark, it automatically enlarges.

* *Accommodation.* This process occurs when the curvature of the lens of your baby's eye varies so that he can focus more clearly. This develops most rapidly during your baby's first three months.

* *Convergence.* In order to focus with single vision on something that is very close, your baby needs to turn both eyes inward at the same time. Convergence steadily develops in the early months.

* *Divergence.* The opposite of convergence, divergence is your baby's ability to focus on a distant object by turning both eyes outward at the same time. Divergence typically develops at the same rate as convergence.

* *Saccades.* When your baby looks around him, his eyes move in very small jerky amounts as he gradually scans his surroundings. The rate at which he is able to do this improves very quickly between birth and four or five months.

* *Visual tracking.* You'll notice that your infant watches an object as it slowly moves across the room. Known as "visual tracking," this ability is present almost at birth and improves steadily over the next few months.

What your baby sees

Researchers have studied the way children under the age of one year use these visual skills to see, and they have found that the

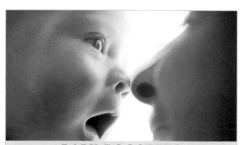

BABY BOOSTERS
COME IN CLOSE

Right from the start your baby is able to focus on an object that is between eight and 15 inches away from her face – this means that your baby is able to see your face during feeding. However, her distance vision is not so good. Make sure, therefore, if you want to catch your baby's interest that you hold your face or toys close to your baby.

typical baby perceives a lot more than most people expect. For example, a newborn baby can tell the difference between a dark image and a light image, and in particular can spot the point where dark and light join. Although not very good at this at birth, your baby makes speedy progress at detecting contours up to the age of six months and then makes slow, steady progress after that.

Newborns see primarily in black and white; the color cells at the back of their eyes – cones, which detect light of different wavelengths – although active at birth, are not fully mature. By three months, however, your baby sees several basic colors (such as red), and by four months, his color vision is fully mature.

In order to see a pattern, the eyes need to inspect and scan all the components of the image, including the edges, center, and overall appearance. Under two months of age, your baby tends to focus mainly on the outer edges and is not good at scanning the whole image. However, this improves in subsequent months.

Aiding your child's progress

Although the world is a constant source of excitement and interest for your growing baby, he faces a particular problem, especially in the early months; he can't easily position himself in order to have the best line of sight. Of course he twists and turns as best he can when he wants to see something, but that can only work to some extent. Until he crawls and sits up on his own, he depends on you to place him in a suitable position for viewing his surroundings, whether he is in his crib, infant seat, or stroller. While riding in the

car he must be rear-facing at all times, but use other opportunities to make sure that he sits in a way that lets him have a good look at all that is going on around him.

Tracking skills

Right from birth your new baby tries to watch or "track" objects as they move around. This visual skill helps him understand what goes on around him; later on it will keep him safe, for instance, as he tracks the movement of cars before crossing the road.

Tracking develops steadily during the early months. Your three-month-old baby can follow slowly an object across the room with his eyes. By the time his first birthday has passed, however, he is easily able to watch you closely as you move around the room. And from nine months on, if he drops something from his hand while sitting in his high chair, he combines his more mature visual tracking skills with his improving memory so that he looks for the fallen object in the correct spot where it fell (see page 78).

Tracking continues to improve so that by that age of three or four years, your child can watch a ball rolling toward him and then put his hands out to scoop it up exactly when it reaches him.

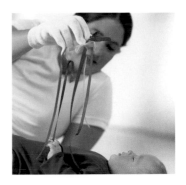

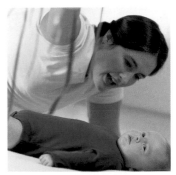

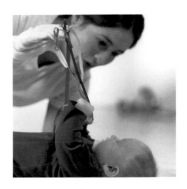

Slowly does It
A young baby can track an object only if it is moved very slowly right in front of her. She isn't mature enough to process visual information at a fast rate and she doesn't have sufficient control over her eye muscles. It also helps if the object is brightly colored or otherwise attracts her attention.

Changes in visual scanning

The way your child uses his visual skills changes as he grows. It goes from:

* *Passive to active.* When he was younger, he looked at something only when it came into his line of vision – he didn't actively search for things to stare at. By age four or five years, however, he consciously chooses what to look at and actively peers at his surroundings until he finds something of interest.

* *Unsystematic to systematic.* When he was an infant, your baby visually scanned a toy haphazardly, perhaps looking at one end, then chewing the opposite end, and so on, without having a specific system to his explorations. At age four or five, he scans his environment more methodically.

* *Broad to selective.* As a young baby, he didn't know where to look when there were two or three things that attracted his attention at the same time. He wasn't very good at filtering out information. Within a few years, however, he is able to focus his visual attention more effectively, so he can look at one item instead of others.

Distance perception

From the moment your infant starts to move around the room, he needs to be able to judge the distance of objects – this helps him to avoid bumping into tables and chairs, enables him to move out of the way when someone approaches, and allows him to reach out accurately toward an object. Depth perception involves:

* *Binocular information.* When you stare at an item, you receive a different image in each eye. When the object is far away, the images are quite similar, and when it is close they are quite different.

* *Interposition information.* You know that when you see one object in front of another, that object is nearer to you than the one it is blocking. Similarly, smaller objects in the distance appear farther away than larger objects.

Your baby doesn't even begin to develop distance vision until at least two months of age and it isn't well established until at least six months.

How vision develops

* *At 2 months:* A baby recognizes his parents' faces and responds with a smile or arm movement. Defensive blink may appear.

* *At 10–12 weeks:* He follows attentively a slowly moving ball held 6–10 inches from his face.

* *At 2–3 months:* Your baby notices some details such as whether pictures are held horizontally or vertically, whether they have single or multiple things on them, and can notice patterns. He watches movements of his own hands and converges his eyes for finger-play. If bottle-fed, a baby recognizes his bottle and

makes eager, welcoming movements as it approaches his face. He spends time staring at distant objects like the furniture across the room or outside the window.

* **At 4–6 months:** Babies are visually very interested, moving head and eyes when activity is perceived. They can discriminate between different emotions such as joy, fear, or sadness and make appropriate responses. Your baby will reach for toys; he will grasp them firmly and observe them closely. Both eyes work together. He can distinguish more subtle shades of colors but may prefer red or blue.

* **At 7–12 months:** Your baby starts to perceive objects as being permanent (see page 78). He will adjust his position to see certain things more clearly. He will look for fallen and hidden toys if he sees them fall while playing with them.

* **At 1 year:** Babies can follow moving objects and see them clearly. They look in the correct places for objects that roll out of sight and recognize familiar people from 20 feet or more. They watch movements of people, animals, and things – indoors and out – with great interest.

TIME FOR A CHECK-UP

Although his vision will be regularly assessed, you should inform your pediatrician if your child:

- Seldom looks at objects in the distance or to the side.
- Looks mostly at objects that are close.
- Appears cross-eyed (eyes that don't move together) after 3 months of age.

PARENTAL PARTICIPATION

By being sensitive to the stage of your baby's visual development, you can ensure that she will get more enjoyment and stimulation from the games you play.

Be a clown

Change your facial expression in an exaggerated way when talking to your baby. She stares at you intently as you feed her or play with her and making your smiles and frowns more emphasized than usual encourages her to develop visual skills.

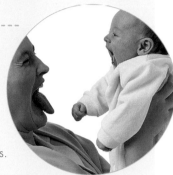

Bright and colorful

When offering toys, remember that simple bright colors are easier for your baby to see. Use red, green, blue, and yellow in preference to more subdued shades.

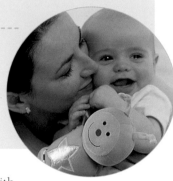

* **At 15–18 months:** Toddlers look with interest at colored pictures in books and touch pages. Can retrieve rolling balls.

* **At 2 years:** Your child has increased interest in objects at distances; vision is more sensitive in the margins of the eye so he may become more distracted. He'll thumb through picture books and will look closely at objects he makes with clay.

* **At 3 years:** Your child shows greater interest in storybook pictures. He can easily follow a moving object and can look without staring. He can copy a circle.

* **At 4 years:** With one eye covered, he can still pick up small items like beads. He can copy a cross. He can name four colors.

object permanence

Child psychologists use the term "object permanence" to refer to the understanding that an object still exists even though it is not directly visible. For instance, you know that if a bottle is put out of sight in a cupboard, you'll be able to open the cupboard door and bring it back out. But that awareness isn't present in young children.

During her first few months, your baby believes the world consists of only the things she can see, so when you leave the room, for example, she assumes you have vanished and when she drops her rattle accidentally, the chances are that she won't look for it. She believes the rattle is no longer in existence because she can't actually see it; for her, it's a case of out of sight, out of mind.

An eight-month-old baby, on the other hand, if shown a toy subsequently hidden by a screen, knows that the toy is still there and will try to push the screen away. And at around nine to 10 months, she will lift a covering to reveal a hidden toy. However, she will continue to look in that same place for the toy even if you've moved it somewhere else.

Nine-month-old babies who engage in repetitive activities such as putting a toy in a box, tipping the box over, picking up the toy, and then replacing it, may be engaging in a version of hide-and-seek and testing the notion of object permanence.

At 10 months, your baby should be able to recognize an object, such as a spoon, if she sees only part of it; in this case, she'll grasp the spoon and put it into her mouth immediately.

Peekaboo games are great ways to help your child learn about object permanence.

During her second year, your child will easily monitor the progress of objects being moved and will be able to find something even if you "hide" it somewhere in sight. She will even look for something she only "suspects" was hidden; she won't

Now you see it...
At seven months a baby will soon "forget" about a toy he's just been playing with if it's covered with a cloth, but by nine to 10 months, he'll lift a covering to reveal a hidden item.

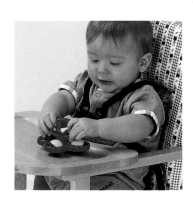
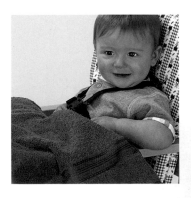
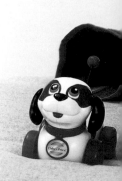

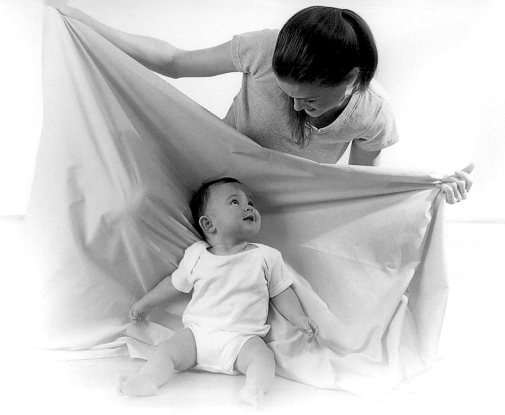

Peekaboo
From a few months old, you can play hide-and-seek games with your baby, but once she's eight or nine months, she won't worry that you might not be there when you lift the covering!

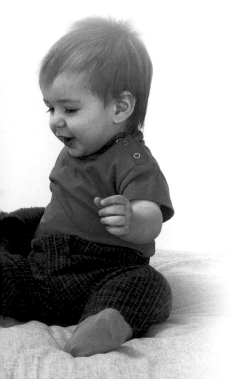

have actually seen the object, only the hand moving something.

The ability to trace objects in space and time, despite their momentary disappearance, is crucial to understanding the way the physical and social worlds behave. It's vital for a baby's stability to realize that you will return even if you are not in the room at that moment. Separation anxiety, when your baby fusses and cries when you leave the room, in large part has to do with your baby not understanding that you'll be back, so keeping in voice contact your baby who can't see you will be reassuring to her. One sign your baby has understood the concept is when she waves "bye-bye" as you go out of the door, beginning at about nine months of age.

An appreciation of object permanence, coupled with the knowledge babies pick up over time about the way things look – their size, texture, shape, and color – helps them to determine the behavior of objects. For example, a baby will soon come to expect all round objects, such as balls, to roll, and the steeper the surface, the faster they'll go.

hearing and listening

Hearing is one of your baby's most important senses; he learns a great deal about the world around him from sounds alone. Massive amounts of information are absorbed through hearing, and this helps his all-around development. A young baby, for example, hears your footsteps approaching, listens to the words you say to him even though he cannot yet speak, has great pleasure listening to music, and may even fall asleep to the continuous sounds of a vacuum cleaner!

Recording of brain waves from the developing fetus confirms that the human hearing system is responsive from around 25 weeks after conception. In other words, your baby's hearing system is up and running months before he is even born.

Once born, babies vary in the sensitivity of their hearing. One newborn might be easily startled and distressed by a loud noise, while another might have a more relaxed attitude. Your baby's individual personality plays a part. However, all new babies typically prefer sounds of a lower frequency to those of a high frequency. Whereas a low tone is likely to calm and relax your baby, a high tone is likely to distress him, perhaps even make him burst into tears. Newborns also show a strong preference for the sound of human voices whether speaking or singing. Most fussy babies can be soothed by noise – lullabies, reassuring words, or the rhythm of a metronome.

How hearing develops

Although your baby can hear right away, it's his degree of selectivity – of recognizing that noise means something and of listening to what he hears – that needs developing. Reaction time to noise also develops over time. A newborn has a much slower reaction to sound than an older child or adult.

* *At birth:* Your baby exhibits the startle or Moro reflex – throwing out arms and legs – in response to loud noise.

* *Around 1½–2 months:* Your baby makes cooing sounds. Looks at a speaker's mouth with interest and responds by smiling.

* *Around 4 months:* Your baby quiets down when he hears your voice, even if he can't see you. He turns his head to a nearby voice. He starts to laugh aloud.

* *Around 6 months:* Although easily distractible, your baby is starting to become more selective to sound. As long as he is not preoccupied with a toy when he hears your voice, he will turn his head immediately to where you are and may turn to listen to quieter sounds made nearby. He may imitate some sounds, shout to attract attention, and vocalize frequently or babble using single and double syllables.

* *Around 9 months:* Your baby may recognize some words, such as his name and "No," by stopping or hesitating during an activity, or waving "bye-bye." He may

appear to listen to others' conversations. He will respond to his name and babble in a string of syllables.

✳ *Around 10 months:* Your baby will probably listen to other people talking and not be distracted by other sounds. He will typically stop what he is doing when he hears "No."

✳ *Around 1 year:* Your baby is able to maintain his interest for longer when he hears someone talking and can look and listen at the same time. His ability to localize sounds is almost as good as an adult. When asked, he may give a toy or other object to you.

✳ *Around 15 months:* Your baby uses a few recognizable words in correct context ("drink milk"). He obeys simple instructions and can find one body part.

✳ *Around 18 months to 2 years:* He's like a sponge when it comes to listening in to other conversations. He can name pictures of common objects. Attends to spoken communications addressed directly to him and may echo prominent or last word in a sentence.

✳ *At 2 years:* Your toddler understands many words, uses two-word phrases, and can follow two-step commands ("Find Teddy. Bring him here."). He knows many body parts and will refer to himself by name.

✳ *At 3 years:* Your child listens eagerly to stories and wants to hear his favorites repeated. He speaks in three-word sentences.

✳ *At 4 years:* Your child listens to and tells long stories; enjoys jokes.

✳ *By 4½ years:* Your child's grammar is usually correct.

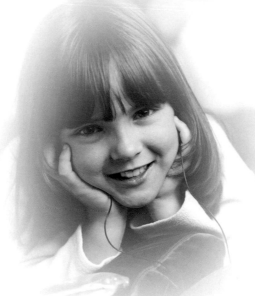

Music lover
Children of all ages like listening to music but only let your older child use headphones and make sure the music isn't too loud and that she doesn't listen for too long.

Aiding your child's progress

The best way to encourage your baby's hearing skills is by providing a range of interesting sounds in his environment. For a start, he likes listening to music, whether on CD or radio, so play a variety, including modern and classical music, and children's songs and rhymes. Sometimes you will notice he kicks his arms and legs in the air in excitement, while other times the music lulls him to sleep! You may find that he suddenly becomes attentive to a sound that you take for granted, such as water gurgling down the drain or a cork being pulled out of a bottle.

Talking to your baby is also critically important. He loves to see your face, hear your voice, and to have your attention, and there is probably no better way to encourage him to use his hearing skills than to speak to him lovingly and enthusiastically. Listening to you also helps him link sounds, facial expressions, body language, and emotions – he learns about lots of different aspects of communication and language just from hearing you speak to him.

Parents often talk instinctively to their baby using "parentese" – shorter sentences,

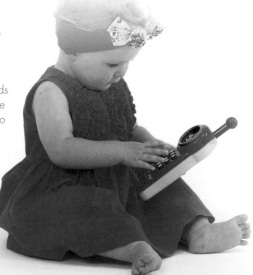

TIME FOR A CHECK-UP

Your baby's hearing will be routinely screened in the newborn nursery, but you should know some of the early-warning signs yourself. See your pediatrician if your baby:

- Doesn't react to loud noise.
- Doesn't turn toward you when you speak to him by four months of age.
- Is startled when he sees you (because he didn't hear your footsteps).
- Doesn't make a range of sounds.
- Won't be soothed by your voice alone.
- Doesn't respond to the sound of a bell gently ringing at his ear.

The earlier a hearing loss is detected, the earlier that help can be given, and the less impact the hearing loss will have on your infant's development.

Rrrrrring
Give your baby a toy that makes a noise when she handles it. This could be a rattle, a cuddly toy that squeaks, or a push-button toy that makes several different sounds when it's touched. She will love being able to make the sounds appear.

smaller words, and exaggerated tones and gestures. Research shows that young babies and infants respond well to this form of language (see also page 104).

Don't forget to read to your baby every day. It's never too early to start and reading out loud is one of the most important things you can do for him. He'll love the sound of your voice, the way in which you change your tone in line with the story's content, and the alteration in facial expression when you reach an exciting part. Hold him in a position that enables him to see the pictures as you point to them, as that helps him develop a link between words and books.

Listening

Never underestimate your child's ability to listen to what he hears – though there is a big difference between the speech and language your child produces himself (this is known as "expressive language") and the language he is able to hear and understand (this is known as "receptive language").

Early on, your growing child understands a lot more than he can say. Although his spoken vocabulary may be limited, he understands many common, everyday words you use – you can tell this by his reaction when you say them to him. Your child grasps the meaning of some sentences that he hears despite the fact he can't speak these same words and sentences himself.

Selective listening

You'll find it amazing, however, that your three-year-old won't hear you when you ask him to put his toys away or get ready for bed, and yet he hears the start of his favorite song. Psychologists call this "selective listening," because in many instances, a child is making a subconscious choice not to respond; he inadvertently chooses to react to some things that he hears and to ignore others.

You won't find it easy to decide whether your child shuts you out using the subconscious process of selective attention or whether, in fact, he is focusing so hard on something else that nothing can penetrate his sound barrier. Resist the temptation to automatically assume that he is subconsciously choosing to zone you out.

Improving listening skills

There are a number of things you can do to improve your child's ability to listen and to concentrate, which he'll need to do to succeed later on in school.

The more distractions surrounding your child, the less likely he is to tune in to your comments. Background noise drowns out the sound of your voice, and also draws his attention to many different directions at once. So if you want him to focus on you, eliminate any distractions, for example, turn down the sound on the television set or CD player. Encourage your child to look at you when you talk to him. Eye contact reduces distractions, allows your child's attention to be more focused, strengthens his concentration, and leads to better understanding.

Your child has an instinctive reaction to turn around when he hears his name. When you want him to listen to you, say his name clearly and loudly, then pause for a moment or two before continuing with what you want to say to him. He needs these few moments to refocus his attention onto you.

Your child will hear you more easily when you are close to him, compared to when you are farther away. Many parents shout when trying to attract their child's attention rather than stop what they are doing and go over to the child. Your child is more likely to hear, understand, and respond to you when you are face-to-face.

PARENTAL PARTICIPATION

No matter how bright and alert he is, your growing child won't learn unless he can listen and concentrate. The ability to concentrate underlies all learning – a child who isn't good at listening takes longer to absorb new ideas and concepts, and needs more time to complete activities.

Read stories

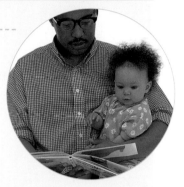

Your child loves the experience of one-on-one storytelling, in which you and he spend time together, close to each other. He concentrates on a story for longer when he enjoys the storytelling context.

Play memory games

For instance, turn four pairs of playing cards facedown on a table. Then ask your child to turn over two cards at a time to find a matching pair. If two different cards are chosen, they are turned facedown again.

Seek and find

Encourage your child to find specific items such as a loaf of bread when shopping in the supermarket or a particular magazine somewhere in the house. Tell him to search for it systematically from room to room, rather than scanning haphazardly.

Teach him songs

Your child may concentrate more on a song when he knows that you expect him to learn the words gradually. Start by asking him to learn the first word of each line and then build up from there.

taste and smell

Taste buds start to appear in your baby's mouth from the eighth week following conception, so her sense of taste is present long before she arrives in the world. Tastes and flavors in your diet during pregnancy are transmitted to your unborn baby through amniotic fluid. Scientists believe this helps your baby recognize you once she is born, as she detects the same tastes in your breast milk. Smell develops early, too, and she is also sensitive to your smell at birth.

Your baby's mouth and tongue are sensitive to touch and taste. Most babies prefer sweet tastes to sour tastes right from birth – your baby will happily gulp down a sweetened drink but turns away from, or spits out, anything that tastes bitter or sour. When she's older and on solids, different foods will have the ability to interest your child more than others. Crunchy and sweet, salty and sour or bitter foods will awaken her taste buds more than mashed or bland foods.

Feeding reflexes
Your baby is also born with reflexes, which enable her to eat and drink. If you gently stroke the side of her cheek, she will stop what she is doing and turn her open lips toward your finger. She may even start moving her mouth.

The moment any food or feeding object (breast or bottle) finds its way into your baby's mouth, she begins to use her mouth and tongue together in order to suck.

As soon as the sucking reflex pushes food from the front of her mouth toward your baby's throat, the swallowing reflex kicks in, allowing her to swallow without choking. It's amazing that these reflexes are

so well coordinated. Without them, your baby couldn't thrive.

Interesting smells
Your baby's sense of taste and smell are interconnected. Sensitivity to your smell – and to the smell of your breast milk if you are feeding her yourself – is present within an hour of her being born! This is another reason why holding your baby against you has such a soothing effect on her. Smell, therefore, helps her bond with you.

As with taste, your baby has smell preferences, which will typically match the smells you like and dislike. For instance, she reacts favorably to sweet, milky, and fruit smells (she smiles, breathes more deeply, relaxes), and reacts adversely to foul smells (kicks her legs, changes her rate of breathing, cries). A strong smell can interfere with her taste; for example, she might not feed so well if you are wearing a very strong perfume.

As your baby gets older, she may become excited about eating when she smells food being prepared. She may bounce in her chair, point, smile, or make noise. However, she also can reject food because of its smell.

mouthing

The world is a fascinating place, as far as your young baby is concerned, and he wants to explore everything he sees, smells, hears, and touches. Every new toy, household object, piece of paper, or item of clothing fills him with excitement, triggering his desire to explore. And one of the best ways for your baby to discover the qualities of an item is by putting it in his mouth.

Your baby's lips and tongue are extremely sensitive and provide him with lots of information. That's why you find that your baby puts objects into his mouth at every opportunity. It's not that he is naughty, disobedient, or challenging, it's just that he wants to know more about these objects, including what they taste like!

During the first six months of life mouthing is your infant's primary means of exploration. Trial and error teaches him that certain items are more suitable for mouthing than others – babies prefer light, plastic, or squishy objects to fuzzy or furry toys – but he may also attempt to mouth large objects too heavy to lift, like a feeding tray, by bending down and sucking on it.

Mouthing hazards

To your baby, a toy looks exciting no matter what condition it is in. Therefore, he is as happy to pop a dirty, dusty object into his mouth as a clean one. Neither will your infant realize the potential dangers that could arise from, say, biting a piece of electrical wire. All he is interested in is the appearance of the item; this means he can easily injure his mouth on a sharp object. He also will try to swallow anything put into his mouth, regardless of size, and

buttons, marbles, and other small items can cause him to choke. Because of this, you must pay special attention to the toys you give him (see page 89). Always look at a toy from your infant's point of view and imagine what would happen if he mouths it.

Using mouthing positively

As mouthing objects is one of the methods your growing baby uses to promote his learning, use it to your advantage. Steer him toward something that will improve his understanding. For instance, he learns more from mouthing a toy when it has interesting and varied textures, when it is easy for him to hold and to bring up to his mouth, and when his chewing is rewarded by a noise or maybe even lights. These features will encourage him to continue with his oral explorations. Since your baby's desire to mouth stems from a genuine need to explore, there is no point in scolding him. Instead, if he's reached for something dangerous or dirty, intervene quickly so that he cannot cause any harm to himself, and direct his attention to a different toy or activity. Always keep unsafe objects out of your child's reach.

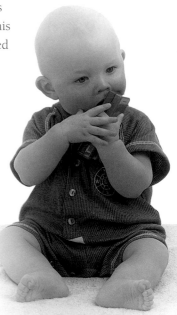

Baby at work
Putting things into his mouth is a great way for your child to learn. The mouth is usually more sensitive than the fingers at this stage, and can teach him a lot about an object's qualities.

touching

Touch is another of the major senses that your baby uses to explore her world. Very early on in life, she acquires some "touch abilities" that help her make new discoveries every day. Touch is also how you first communicate with your baby while feeding, holding, bathing, and cuddling her. Nothing soothes a newborn quite so much as her nestling skin to skin against her parent.

Teaching tool
What your baby learns about an object through her sense of touch influences the way she reaches for or grasps it.

Research studies confirm that touch sensation begins in the womb and that as a newborn, your baby's skin is very sensitive. Scientists have discovered an embryo is responsive to touch from about seven or eight weeks after conception. Once she's born, a baby reacts to a puff of air on her skin, even when the force of that puff is so slight that you would barely feel it. A newborn also exhibits the grasp reflex

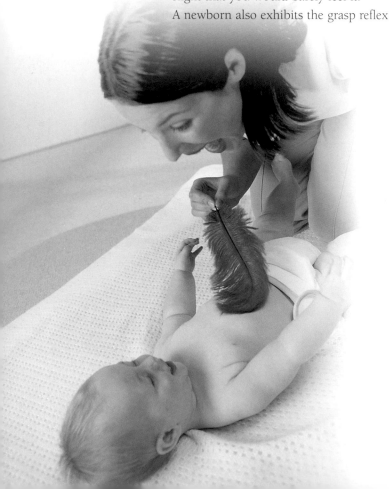

(when you stroke your baby's palm she'll curl her fingers to grip yours) and is able to grip an object very tightly when it is placed into the palm of her hand.

The development of touch

Touch in combination with hearing and vision refines fine motor skills and enables your new baby to reach out for objects that attract her attention. Although reaching appears a simple task, it's actually quite complex. That's why for the first few months, an infant's reaching strategy is ineffective – her hand either closes before it gets to the object or it closes after, in each instance making it impossible for her to grab hold of the item.

By the age of four to five months, however, your growing infant's reaching ability becomes more effective and the evolving coordination of looking, reaching, and grasping, gives her newfound opportunities to discover and learn.

These, in turn, can lead to the development of likes and dislikes. Most babies and toddlers enjoy feeling different textures with both their hands and feet – and many young baby toys are made up of a variety of different materials – and they develop preferences for certain touch sensations. However, your baby also may suddenly develop a strong dislike for certain textures; many children, for example, don't like the feel of sand or mud on their feet, or food that is too cold or hot.

The stages in acquiring touch

As with the other senses, touch develops mainly over the course of your baby's first year.

* *Around 3 months:* With her hands opened more, your baby enjoys feeling something placed in her hand and notices the difference between soft and hard.

* *Around 4 months:* Your baby can now bring her hands to midline and use her fingers for active exploration. Mouthing becomes more important; as soon as she grasps something, into her mouth it goes.

* *Around 5 months:* Splashing in the bath may become an enjoyable activity.

* *Around 6 months:* Now more than ever, your baby prefers toys that she can interact with and listen to as well as things she can touch.

* *Around 7–8 months:* Your baby is beginning to learn about spatial relationships, the difference between flat and round objects, what's on the top and what's on the bottom. Enjoys objects with grabable parts, such a labels, handles, and strings.

* *Around 9–10 months:* Object permanence (see page 78) becomes established. Your baby can handle toys more appropriately, taking into account the special properties of objects such as shaking a rattle, putting a cup to her mouth, or crinkling pieces of tissue paper. She will enjoy feeding herself with her fingers.

PARENTAL PARTICIPATION

Tactile input (feeling) is very important to your baby's development. It is one of the ways she integrates sensory behavior and forms a concept of her body. There are various ways you can provide tactile experiences.

Baby massage

Early physical contact is very important to your baby. Gentle stroking and rubbing of your baby's body on a regular basis from an early age can calm and reassure your baby and directly express the love you feel for her.

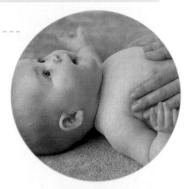

Expand her consciousness

Keeping safety in mind, encourage your baby to experience different sensations; for example, have her walk without shoes on carpet, tile, and wood; let her feel feathers, fur, and fabric. Under supervision, allow her to play with water, sand, and clay.

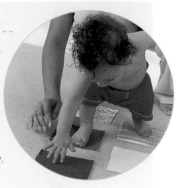

* *Around 10–11 months:* Your baby is learning concepts such as behind or inside; she likes poking her fingers into holes and tearing paper. Tactile likes and dislikes may become more apparent.

* *Around 12 months:* She enjoys experimenting with all textures – sticky, slimy, hard, cold, squishy, etc.

play for the senses

No matter how old they are, children love to play, and it is through play that they develop their skills. It is not always necessary to buy toys for a child and, particularly in the early years, simple, safe objects found around the house and homemade toys will be great sources of entertainment.

Books

It is never too early to start to look at books with your child. Set aside time every day to read. Your baby will enjoy cuddling up to you, listening to the sound of your voice while you page through a book together. However, it is from six months or so that children really start to become interested in books, particularly those with large bright pictures and simple stories. As they get older, they will come to enjoy the surprises of lift-the-flap and pop-up books. They will also enjoy playing with waterproof picture books in the bath.

Sand play

Popular with all young children, they love pouring, digging, and shaping sand. You don't need a sand pit. Buy a small sack of child-friendly sand and decant it into a plastic box. Add plastic pails and shovels, sieve, digger, and tractor. Older children will enjoy weighing the sand with a set of simple

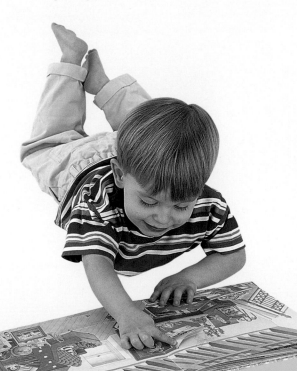

TOP TOYS

Age recommendations printed on toy packages are important. They reflect safety aspects and developmental levels for various age groups.

- **1–3 months:** Rattles, mobiles, bright board books with bold colors.
- **4–7 months:** Textured toys that make sounds; baby mirror; baby books with board or vinyl pages.
- **8–12 months:** Stacking toys; bath toys; large building blocks; push-pull toys; "busy boxes" that push, open, and squeak.
- **13–18 months:** Lift-out puzzles; digging toys; cars, trucks, and trains; board books; shape sorters; dolls; crayons.
- **19 months–2 years:** Hammering toy; simple puzzles; toy telephone; musical toys.
- **2–3½ years:** Construction toys; dress up clothes; paints; toy tools and safe household items (i.e. dustpan and brush).
- **3½–5 years:** Magnetic boards; sport toys; music player; pop-up books.

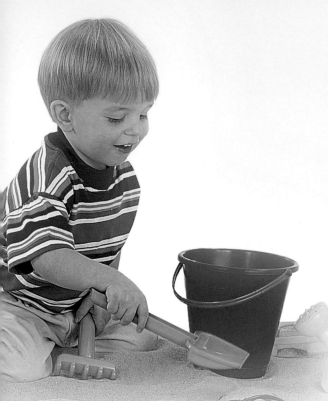

scales. Wet sand also is great fun; give your child jello molds and small plastic containers for shaping the sand.

Water play

Supervised time playing with water is great fun for your child both indoors and out. Whether splashing in the bath, frolicking under a hose, floating boats in the kitchen sink, or simply blowing bubbles, children find water fascinating. It also provides plenty of opportunities for learning – as long as you keep an eye on your child. Never leave him alone with water.

Give your child beakers with which to measure and pour, toys that float or sink, or let him wash his own tea set or play dishes.

Choosing toys

Before you select any toy, ask yourself:

* Is it suitable for my child's developmental stage? In most cases you are really talking about whether a toy is appropriate and safe for a particular age, as most children achieve their milestones around the same age. However, it is also worth thinking about the stage your child has reached in terms of his skills. Is he banging things? Trying to put one object on top of another? Trying to turn knobs? Picking up pens and trying to scribble? You can have great fun looking around for toys that will stimulate your child. Many children's toys are labeled with the appropriate age range. Avoid toys that are likely to be too advanced – your child will either lose interest in them rapidly or become frustrated by them, or might even injure himself on a piece made for an older child.

* Is it safe? Look for toys that appear to be robust and hard-wearing. Avoid toys that look as though they may break or that have sharp edges, small toys that could be swallowed, or toys that have small parts that may be chewed or broken off – either could be a choking hazard. It is also important to avoid toys with strings or cords that are more than six inches long; the danger of strangulation is too great.

* Is it fun? If a toy uses your baby's skills and stimulates his senses, he is likely to find it fun. Avoid trying to speed up your baby's development by forcing toys he is not yet ready for. Let him have fun and develop his skills in his own time. Always keep an eye on what your baby or toddler enjoys playing with at baby groups or your friends' or relatives' houses.

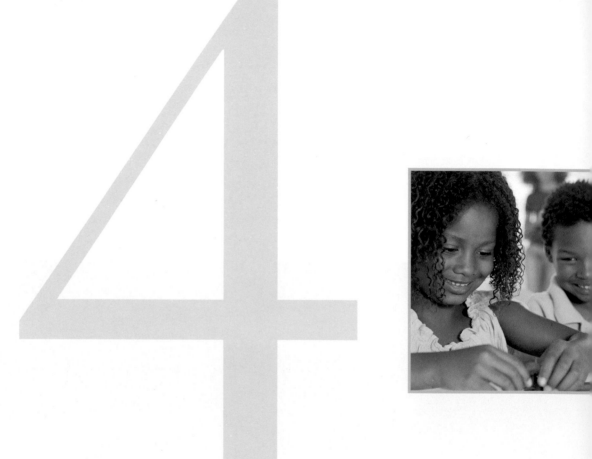

mental development

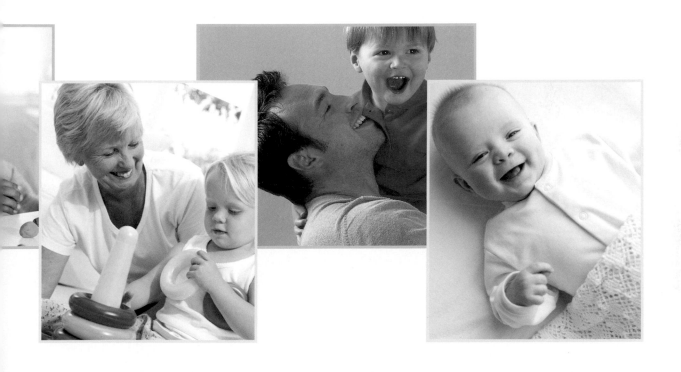

understanding the stages

Your child's mental abilities will develop remarkably between birth and when she reaches school age. Over time she will acquire the ability to interpret the world and to communicate. When she becomes a school-aged student she will be better able to digest complex information, make advanced plans, recall strategies she has used in previous learning tasks, think through problems toward a solution, and communicate solutions and ideas.

What is mental development?

In reality there are many strands to the mind. There is "understanding," or "thinking," often referred to as "cognitive" or "intellectual" development. This concerns reasoning, analysis, and problem solving. It involves first being exposed to something new and then applying this experience to subsequent new and unfamiliar situations. For a newborn baby, the problem may be hunger, and she is likely to learn that a more high-pitched cry produces milk faster than a whimper. For a three-year-old child, the challenge may be how to coax a treat from Granddad, and learning that looking cute and saying "Pleeeease…" in a certain sort of voice has a high chance of yielding the desired result. Clearly, cognition evolves from the simple and concrete to the almost infinitely complex and abstract.

Mental development also involves communication, which consists not only of words but also gestures, facial expressions, cries, and other noises. Sometimes it is about behaviors, such as tantrums. It is about choosing to follow a suggestion (or not), or to obey a command (or not). It is about emotions as well as facts.

"Emotional intelligence" is a term that is used to describe the ability to understand the communication of feelings. There are two aspects to this: One is understanding what is said "between the lines," which means both body language and the way tone of voice may convey something more than words themselves. The other is about the ability to see things from the perspective of another person. Here the type of information to be processed is very different from that mentioned before: it is abstract, yet it is of fundamental importance as children have to learn how to build relationships and friendships. It begins within the first few weeks after birth as infant and parents interact, and continues as children start to imitate others and later to engage in cooperative or collaborative play. Specialists increasingly believe that the development of emotional intelligence comes before the development of reasoning and structured thought.

Perception is a mental function that is fundamental to development. The ability to hear is mature before birth. The ability to see develops rapidly over the first year of life and is mature by the age of five or six. But the way in which the information is handled and processed is, in part, culturally and socially determined. Adults are good at filtering out extraneous information, but young children who have not learned what is to be considered extraneous, attach equal importance to everything that happens within their range of sight or sound. This can appear as difficulty with concentration or easy distractibility to the adult, but to the child it is simply a case of different priorities.

Then there are games. These involve communication, problem solving, facts, and emotions, as well as trust, deception, pretense, and competition. Games are probably critically important for certain kinds of learning, and they also evolve from the very simple and concrete (like peekaboo), to the complex and abstract (simple charades).

These are not the only aspects of mental function that exist, and each can be further subdivided, but they give a flavor of the diversity of aspects of the mind.

The importance of parents

Babies thrive in an environment where they get lots of love and attention. The environment that you create for your baby will influence the way she deals with her emotions, the way she interacts with people, the way she thinks, and the way she grows physically.

By creating an enriching environment for your child, you are allowing normal brain development to take place. This type of environment is one that is "child centered" and provides opportunities for learning that are geared to your child's development, interests, and personality. Fortunately, the components of a good environment include basic things that most parents know and want to provide for their children: Proper nutrition; a warm, responsive, and loving family as well as other caregivers; fun playtime; consistent, positive reinforcement; engaging conversations; good books to read and to listen to; music to stimulate brain activities; and the freedom to explore and learn from their surroundings.

A caring child
The ability to help take care of a pet relates not only to your older child's thinking skills in working out what to do but also her emotional intelligence in anticipating the creature's needs.

Mental development begins before birth and is linked to other types of development, particularly sensory development (see pages 68–89) and the amount of stimulation a child receives. Keep in mind these milestones should only be used as guidelines.

4 weeks:	Hears well. Seems to prefer the sound of mother's voice. May look around to find source of sound; and watches alertly when fed and talked to.
6 weeks:	Smiles at you and coos responsively.
3 months:	Moves fingers at will. Has a variety of sounds and gestures as "conversation." If bottle-fed, recognizes bottle; reacts with excitement to familiar situations such as feeding and bathing.
4 months:	Exhibits curiosity in new things and sensations; may exhibit the beginnings of a sense of humor.
5 months:	Starts to understand simple game playing and spends more time examining things. Smiles at own face in mirror.
6 months:	Makes attention-seeking noises; may raise arms to be picked up. May be shy with strangers and exhibit fear. Grasps and shakes rattle.
8 months:	Begins to understand the meaning of words, particularly "no." Will look for a dropped toy.
9 months:	Recognizes familiar games and rhymes; plays peekaboo. Laughs in appropriate parts. Turns head to name. Distinguishes familiar faces from strangers.
10 months:	Waves bye-bye and pats a doll or stuffed animal. Looks around corners for a toy. Likes to laugh and is interested in books.
1 year:	Says a couple of words. Recognizes certain objects in books and points to them; begins to understand simple questions. Plays pat-a-cake.
15 months:	Can make some animal sounds; knows 4–6 words including names. Has developed certain concepts such as what is a dog and can identify one in a book or at the park. Explores properties of toys.
18 months:	Looks selectively at a book. Can imitate a drawing stroke. May attempt a few chores – will imitate your actions. May follow a simple command. Knows certain parts of body.
21 months:	Can ask for toys, food, and potty. Is beginning to understand more complicated requests. Can fold paper imitatively. Pulls a person to show something.

2 years:	Has a rapidly increasing vocabulary.
	Points to and names familiar objects. Can describe the properties of certain items.
	Obeys complicated orders.
2½ years:	Knows some nursery rhymes and colors.
	Recognizes minute details in picture books.
	Plays meaningfully with toy cars and dolls' house furnishings.
3 years:	Asks questions incessantly.
	Builds complicated structures.
	Can remember the past.
	Knows sex, first and last name.
	Copies a circle.
4 years:	Copies a cross.
	Counts 1–10.
	Matches and names four colors.
	Gives connected account of recent events and experiences.
	Enjoys jokes.
	Appreciates past, present, and future.
5 years:	Counts fingers on one hand.
	Produces pictures containing several items and a background.
	Fluent speech; can learn home address and phone number.
	Plays well alone or with friends.

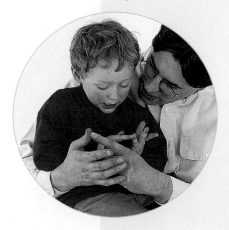

Counting games
Most parents teach their children "their numbers." Grasping numeracy is a long process that begins when a child learns the numbers in order by counting his fingers or objects.

Problems such as maternal depression or disease that cause significant changes in maternal or caregiver behaviors or emotions can interfere with parent-child interaction and have the potential to impact a child's normal development.

The role of a parent or primary caregiver is critically important for healthy child development. Each child, however, brings their own unique temperamental characteristics to the parent-child relationship. Often the pairing of temperament between a parent or caregiver and child can have a strong influence on the child's development.

Parents or primary caregivers also influence the way a baby learns. It is easiest to see this with language because the sounds parents (and others) reflect back to their babies are those that are used linguistically by the parents themselves. Thus reinforcement is acting on the sounds that will later make up the baby's language even as the baby is developing a repertoire of different vocalizations.

Through your communication and interaction with your baby, you and your baby can share feelings as well as needs. There is an increasing consensus of opinion among pediatricians and developmental psychologists that the communication of feelings may be of fundamental importance to all areas of mental development. That is why your baby needs you to be responsive to her, not just for the formation of a long-term attachment but also for her everyday happiness and contentment. Research has shown that babies significantly benefit from regular, frequent, and positive interaction with their primary caregivers.

responding

Babies have an emotional need to form a close, loving emotional attachment with at least one caring adult in their lives. This interactive relationship provides children with a strong foundation, which will aid them throughout childhood and adulthood and can be a strong predictive factor for their responses during times of stress.

We now know that babies respond within the first hour after birth. Through videotaped encounters it is possible to see quite subtle nuances of their mothers' facial expressions and speech eliciting changes of facial expression of their own, and with noises. Over several minutes they may have periods of more or less engagement with their mothers, and sensitive mothers follow these patterns, not pushing for engagement when it is not occurring, but reacting to it and reinforcing it when it does occur. In fact, the movements of mother and baby – head and limbs as well as facial movement – follow each other like dancing partners, alternately initiating and reinforcing the actions of the other.

As a baby grows, his repertoire of responses increases as his basic physical abilities, such as head control, allow for a richer diversity of movements. Parents and other caregivers choose their manner of approach according to the emotional state of the baby, such as whether the baby is looking serious, playful, or distressed.

As you and your baby get to know each other, you're likely to find yourself meshing your responses with each other without even thinking about it. For instance, he cries, you pick him up; he cuddles into you, and you pull him close; he makes cooing noises because he is happy, and you copy his cooing and say soothing words back to him. It's this sensitivity to each other's psychological signals and emotional needs – each of you responding and interacting with the other – that builds and intensifies your relationship.

You should be aware, however, that babies vary in their responsiveness to others right from birth. This means that some parents have to work harder than others when it comes to getting a reaction from their baby. There are two extremes in the level of responsiveness (although most babies are somewhere in between):

* **Active**. These babies are very expressive, and give out very strong and frequent social signals (for example, eye contact, reaching, smiling, and vocalizing).

* **Passive**. These babies have passive facial expressions that reveal nothing about their inner emotions.

You and your baby may not form an instant bond. In many families, the meshing process between parent and child takes weeks or even months, so don't try to rush it: It will happen naturally if you give each other time. Your baby's instinct is to look at you, tune in to your voice, and snuggle up against you. He doesn't need to be told how to get close to you – and you don't need to be told how to act lovingly toward him. Follow your intuition.

Determining responsiveness

A young baby is more responsive to you at some times than at others. There are moments when his eyes are fully open and he is wide awake and keen to absorb all that goes on around him; at other points in the day, his eyes are tightly closed and you can hear him breathe heavily. And sometimes you can't actually tell if he is asleep or not! As your baby learns most when he is wide awake and alert, it is important that you get to know his individual habits and sleep patterns – the time when he is most alert is the best time for involving him in stimulating play.

The fact that your baby is awake, however, does not mean he is responsive and ready for stimulation. Other factors influence him, too. For instance, if he lies calmly and quietly in his crib and you approach him, he smiles and perhaps moves his arms and legs with delight; but if he is highly aroused and upset, he doesn't react at all to that sort of stimulation.

Bear in mind, too, that when your baby is playing with toys, moving his hands in front of himself, or making sounds, he is instinctively seeking amusement for himself. He doesn't need your stimulation constantly. In fact, too much stimulation can make him fussy or can make him tune out and become less responsive. You'll soon learn what stimulation works best with your child. You'll find, for instance, that there is no point in showing him a toy

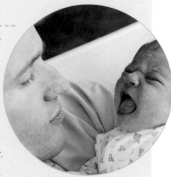
while he is feeding as his concentration is totally focused on eating, whereas singing to him might help the feeding process along. Likewise, you'll learn that perhaps he is most alert either first thing in the morning or early in the evening. As you become familiar with your baby's natural cycles of attention you can adjust your degree of stimulation and involvement.

information processing

The ability to think is referred to as "cognitive ability." Such commonplace terms as "intelligence," "IQ" (intelligence quotient), and "intellectual ability" are often used to measure cognitive ability. In preschool children this can be difficult to measure because the skills required are not yet well developed.

Conceptualizing
Figuring out which of a number of rings is the next one to add may be solved by a process of trial and error or simply by considering the object itself.

Most parents find that by the end of their child's first year they start to have an idea as to how well she remembers people or things. Over the next few years as your child engages in more and more activities, you'll have more opportunity to gain some idea of how quickly your child learns, and how well the learning is remembered.

Skill building

The development of children's learning skills (also known as "thinking skills," "cognitive skills," "intellectual skills," and "mental skills") involves several different dimensions, including:

* *Problem solving.* When babies are confronted with a problem they have limited ideas on how to solve it. In contrast, five-year-olds will consider many possibilities and then test them out through trial and error striving for success.

* *Concentration.* A young baby's ability to concentrate is fairly limited; she darts from one thing to another very easily. An older child learns to focus on a game until the end point is reached, or until the challenge is tackled effectively.

- - - - - - - - - - - - - - - - - -

In the know... *Early IQ*
The only ability in young children that bears much relation to cognition is the rate at which speech and language are acquired – and even this does not relate all that well to later intelligence.

- - - - - - - - - - - - - - - - - -

* **Memory.** During childhood, memory improves with age. A young baby's recall is limited and is confined to objects or people she sees every day, unlike when she's older and she'll be able to recall information she learned days, weeks, or months before.

* **Symbolic thought.** Under the age of one, children typically think about what they see in front of them. During the second year they begin to think about matters in their heads, without having to actually see things. This is the emergence of symbolic thought.

* **Inquisitiveness.** A baby has a limited ability to explore and gain information. At five years old, however, she is able to ask questions in order to satisfy her thirst for knowledge – this enables her to acquire vast amounts of information from others.

Thinking styles

Each child approaches learning differently. Similarly with responsiveness (see page 96), psychologists have identified two main styles, with the majority of children falling somewhere along the continuum.

If your child spends a great deal of time thinking and planning before she actually does anything, she has what's known as a reflective learning style. She imagines various different possibilities in her mind and runs through these, carefully weighing up the pros and cons. Only when she feels confident does she try out her ideas in practice. A reflective learning style involves patience, planning skills, and the ability to wait.

On the other hand, if your child immediately flies at a problem with great enthusiasm, preferring to discover as she goes along, she has what's called an impulsive approach. She is not particularly troubled by early failures – she learns from these as they occur and quickly moves on. Before the child with the reflective style has lifted a finger, the impulsive learner has tested out several different solutions.

Each learning style has its own advantages. For instance, a reflective style is useful when there is plenty of time and there can only be one attempt at finding a solution, whereas an impulsive learning approach is useful when time is short and a solution is needed quickly. Your child probably shows elements of both learning styles at different times.

The processes of thinking

The most popular psychological theory of mental development is that a child uses mental "schemes" to represent, organize, and understand her experiences. A baby starts off with a few very basic schemes for making sense of her surroundings but these gradually extend as she grows older. A child's schemes – and therefore her mental development – change as a result of three processes.

When a child learns new information she fits it into her existing schemata. For example, if your two-year-old already is familiar with the concept of "dog" and sees another animal with four legs, such as a horse, she thinks it could be a dog, too. She uses her existing schema for "dog" and assimilates the image of the horse into it.

However, your child is also able to change her existing schemata on the basis of new information. Suppose she sees the horse and realizes that although it has four legs like a dog, it is a different size, with

PARENTAL PARTICIPATION

Memory builders

You can help develop your child's memory by reminding her of what she did before – talking over incidences and experiences – and by playing matching games where she has to recognize common objects.

Have fun with numbers

Incorporate numbers into everything you do; count items when you shop, the pieces of a game, the clothing your child puts on.

Look for patterns

All kinds of patterns – visual, auditory, and motor – can be found in your child's world. Encourage her to tune in to these patterns by drawing her attention to things that appear in the landscape, can be heard in songs and speech, and can be followed, such as fitting puzzle pieces together.

different hair, a longer tail, and so on. As a result, she accommodates her new learning by increasing her existing schemata so that now there is one for dogs and another one for horses.

Your growing child has an emotional need for her world to stay in balance, to have a settled understanding of the world around her. She constantly modifies her mental development as she learns, in order to maintain this equilibration. The whole motivation of curiosity is that she is able to makes sense of something she doesn't understand in order to regain her sense of balance.

Aiding your child's progress

One of the most useful approaches during childhood for improving your child's learning capacity and thinking skills is "scaffolding." In the same way that builders construct a temporary structure to use as a platform for building a more permanent one, intellectual scaffolding can be used with children to help them move from one level of understanding to another. Suppose, for instance, your three-year-old has a jigsaw that she cannot solve, and doesn't even know how to start. You might show her how to pick out the four corners first and then to find the joining pieces. That help might be all she needs to solve the rest of the puzzle, too. By providing that "scaffold" of learning for your child, you help her reach new learning heights. You'll find that you can gradually reduce the level of scaffolding until she reaches the point where she is an independent learner.

communication

Your child communicates with you verbally (for instance, by using cries, spoken sounds, and words) and nonverbally (for instance, by using facial expression, head and body movements, arm and leg movements, and eye contact). Communication is a two-way process, no matter your child's age – it involves an exchange of feelings and ideas, passing back and forth between you.

How communication skills develop

* **At birth:** Your baby's main form of communication is usually expressed by crying – that's how he lets you know that he may be unhappy, hungry, or in pain. He also uses facial gestures and body movements to communicate his feelings.

* **By 3 months:** He may have picked up that crying is a good way to grab your attention, and he begins to understand that his behavior generates a reaction from you (for instance, when he smiles, you smile back).

* **Between 4 and 6 months:** Your baby may begin to use distinctive sets of recognizable speech sounds, such as "m" or "b" – he tends to repeat the same sound in quick succession. It looks as if he is trying to talk to you with his babbling sounds.

* **At 6 months:** Although spoken language hasn't appeared, your infant may start to behave as though he understands the social rules of conversation. You'll notice that when you talk, he may stop babbling, and then start again once you stop.

* **By 1 year:** The emergence of your baby's first word around this time – generally "mama" or "dada" – opens a whole new set of communication possibilities for your baby. For the first time, he may use a sound combination (a word) to indicate a specific object.

* **Around 18 months:** Your toddler may now begin to put two or more words together to form a meaningful phrase (for instance, "me milk" to tell you that he wants a drink of milk).

* **At 2 years:** With the increasing ability to talk in phrases or short sentences, your toddler learns the power of the word "no," and uses this emphatically when he wants to stop you from doing something he dislikes. Even though he can speak, he

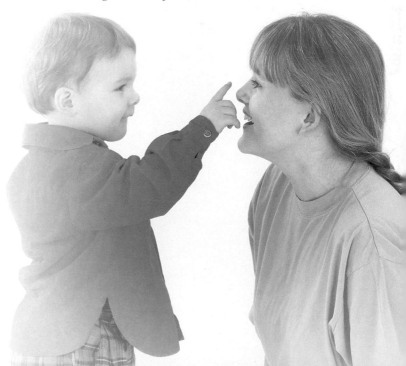

Pointing
Used from an early age, and always as a form of communication, it shows that a baby is able to understand more than he can say.

continues to conveys his feelings non-verbally as well, using a broader range of gestures, such as walking away, clenching his fist, staring directly at someone, and cuddling – you understand what he means even though he may not say a word.

✳ Between 3 and 5 years:
Communication extends rapidly to include others in his world, particularly his friends. He loves chatting to them as they play cooperatively together, exchanging ideas and comments at the same time.

His body language becomes more complex as he combines individual gestures together to make a new meaning. For instance, if he pulls at his ear, his cheeks redden, and his eyes look solidly at his feet, you may suspect this means he is hiding something from you.

✳ At 6 years: With a good range of speech skills, your child is much more effective at giving accounts of incidents, both pleasurable and distressing, to you. He will begin to recognize the emotional benefits of talking things over with others. At this point in his development, your child also may recognize he can use body language deliberately in order to convey his intentions. For example, he smiles at someone whom he wants to play with, or he deliberately frowns and stamps his feet when he wants you to know he is angry.

Crying

From birth on, crying is your baby's dominant sound and its importance cannot be stressed too much. The human baby relies on his parents for food, warmth, and protection; and since looking after babies is hard work, the baby has a vested interest in generating commitment from his parents. Crying creates powerful emotions in parents and any other nearby adult, and adults feel the need to go to the baby and deal with whatever the baby might lack. The way in which a baby cries, particularly the pitch of his cry, is important in promoting the adult's need to help him.

The cry of a particular baby is fairly distinctive, so that many mothers can often (but not always) tell their baby from other babies, by cry alone, within a few days of birth. Some cries also have distinct meanings. There is agreement among researchers that cries can relate to pain, but whether other cries relate distinctively to hunger, anger, or even pleasure is disputed. Many parents develop a sense of when their baby is hungry, angry, in pain, fearful, wanting a diaper change, uncomfortable (too hot or too cold, for instance), or just bored, and the detection of these distinctions increases as the baby gets older. On the other hand, some parents feel that they cannot distinguish between their infants' cries.

Throughout his early years, your child will continue to find crying an important means of expressing extremes of emotion – desire, anger, and frustration – and he may often accompany it with words that try to make the reason for the crying absolutely clear. He might also use crying where words quite literally fail him, yet there is a powerful need to convey a need or feeling.

Vocalizations

But crying is not your young baby's only sound. There are lots of other noises that babies make, although they may take a few weeks to appear, and usually follow the development of social smiling.

Cooing and gurgling start to be heard around the second month. Cooing is a combination of laughter and vowel sounds, and typically tells you that your baby is happy and content. Coos are long strings of the same vowel sound but are more varied than cries, and involve different mouth muscles. Most parents find these sounds very captivating and enjoy spending more time with their baby when he vocalizes in this way. Unlike crying, cooing conveys your baby's positive feelings. Even if the coos at times resemble words, that is purely coincidence; there is no meaning attached to them.

From the third month your baby may expand his repertoire of sounds, including squealing, growling, and blowing raspberries. At the same time, he will start to experiment with consonants. These vocalizations are clearly associated with comfort and discomfort but they are not cries, and therefore do not carry the same message of urgency.

Laughter follows around a month after social smiling, and it evolves out of the cooing and gurgling expressed before. Initially, babies need stimulation by facial and vocal expressions, and touch to elicit laughter, but by five or six months, novel situations or stimuli, which might have caused crying at a younger age, can produce laughter, too. Older siblings often can make a baby laugh easier than an adult. By one year of age, laughter has become a response to many situations such as simple jokes or deceptions.

From about 7 to 10 months of age, babies increasingly make patterns of consonants and vowels (BaBaBa…, DaDaDa…), gradually expanding into

---

In the know... *Influences on babbling*

Evidence suggests that babbling is affected both by nature and nurture. On the nature side, scientists have found that baby babbling tends to be the same, irrespective of the language used by the parents, which suggests there is a biological component to it. On the nurture side, research has shown that babies who do not hear speech (because of hearing loss) don't start babbling till later and have a more restricted range of babbling sounds. In addition, where a baby hasn't had the opportunity to babble, for example, due to having a breathing tube inserted, it takes a long time for him to catch up after the tube is removed. This suggests the environment plays a part, too.

---

different vowel and consonant patterns (BaDa, BaBi).

As he nears the age of 12 months, your infant's babbling is no longer reduplicated and instead he joins different sound units together, for instance, "ba-leh." This more sophisticated form of babbling may remind you in some ways of speech, and you may at times think he is actually talking to you, because he varies his voice tone and his voice pitch rises and falls just like adult speech. You'll also notice that your infant may occasionally use the same babbled sound string in the same context, indicating his understanding that he senses a link between sounds and meaning. Many of the babbling sounds he uses now will eventually form part of his first words.

After the acquisition of their first words, young children continue to experiment with sounds that may or may not be vocal such as whispering, singing, and chanting. Adult reactions to initially involuntary noises such as burping or passing gas often encourage toddlers to imitate these sounds for the entertainment of themselves and others.

Aiding your child's progress

Remember that your young baby quite often uses vocalizations for a purpose. That said, sometimes he makes sounds for the purpose of amusing himself, as a form of play, but other times he babbles for the purpose of connecting with you, of stimulating a reaction from you. Your positive responses to his babbling teach him the value of communication. You'll find that if you talk back to him as if you know what he is trying to tell you, he will stop babbling and listen. That's why psychologists view this verbal interaction between parent and infant as an early type of conversation, which in a few years will evolve into full sentences rather than sounds.

Vocalizations are important because they are the basis of language, as well as being important communications in their own right. As your baby experiments with a wide range of sounds, you will pick up and reflect back to him those sounds that exist in your native language, so that he has positive feedback for making those sounds that will later become his true language.

Bear in mind that children vary greatly in the level of responsiveness to communication. One baby might wriggle and squeal with delight when his parent sings him a song, while another might lie there passively and enjoy the experience. One four-year-old might have a verbal explosion when he comes home from child care because he is so anxious to share his

exciting accounts of what happened there, while another might come home without saying more than a couple of words. These individual differences in communication habits are perfectly normal.

If your child has a quieter nature, don't push him too hard. Give him space and time to say what he has to say to you, when he wants. He'll talk to you when he is ready, not before, and pressing him to

----

In the know... *Parentese*

When talking to a baby, adults commonly use "baby language." This is a phenomenon common to many cultures. One characteristic of this kind of speech is its higher pitch than normal adult speech, with extra stress at the beginnings of words. In addition, they often use a questioning tone, which rises at the end of a phrase, rather than the falling tone that is used with most statements made to other adults. Some adults use "baby" words that imitate the mispronunciations that are characteristic of two- and three-year-old children. Baby language has a simplified structure and a narrowed range of sounds. It specifically arouses and engages babies, and starts a reciprocal "conversation" that may also include touch, lots of eye contact, many varieties of facial expression, and simple games. In turn, babies learn the kind of behaviors that may encourage such attention from nearby adults.

----

speak more could create a barrier between you. In addition, look at his nonverbal behavior – you may be able to tell what sort of mood he is in, what sort of day he has had, by studying his body language closely. You may find that your child goes through phases in which he is more (or less) communicative than he was before.

Nonverbal communication

Your baby can use nonverbal means to pass information to you about his thoughts and feelings. Also known as "body language," it is an important form of communication – as important as spoken language. Interpreting his body language can help you understand your child.

The most important facial communication is the smile. However, even before smiling develops, a tiny baby may choose to make eye contact, will search visually over a face placed in the field of vision, may indicate satiety by refusing more feeding, and may communicate tension or repose by alterations in muscle tone. Although a young baby can't grasp the meaning of words spoken to him and can't take part in a conversation with you, he does interpret the nonverbal signals that accompany your speech, such as your smile, the gentle tone of your voice, and the way you hold him when speaking to him. He responds to these in his own way, perhaps by looking intently in your face, or smiling back at you, or making soft cooing noises to indicate his delight.

Smiling

Smiling is one of the most exciting and important things that a baby does. Once social smiling occurs, it is the start of a new phase because parent and baby can signal positive emotions to each other. Before this, it was the absence of crying, rather than the presence of smiling, that was the closest a baby could come to expressing emotion.

More than 30 years ago it was found that babies gradually build up their capacity to smile. In the first few days, a smile appears in the corners of the mouth. By one week of age, babies will frequently smile in the "active" phase of sleep, when other parts of their bodies may move as well, and this can happen as a response, delayed by several seconds, to low-level sounds such as a human voice. By his second week, more of a baby's mouth is involved and this is often seen after a feeding.

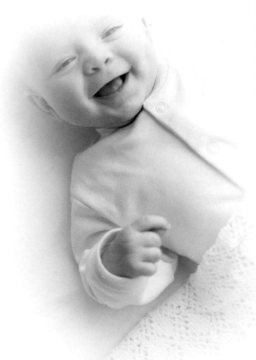

Early smiles
Your baby begins smiling almost from birth – but you will find it hard to detect before six weeks of age. Babies born nearer their expected dates of delivery smile before those born later (or pre-term babies).

Around three weeks, more of the face is involved, especially the eyes, and in response to a wider variety of noises. Babies particularly do this in their quiet wakeful phases, in which they are usually spending increasing amounts of time, and the delay is less – more like four or five seconds. At about a month, this kind of smile can happen because of touch as well as voice, and the smile involves the whole face. Somewhere between five and eight weeks (or more for babies born well before their due dates), true emotionally interactive smiling, just in response to an adult smile, happens for the first time. This is social smiling. At this stage, smiling

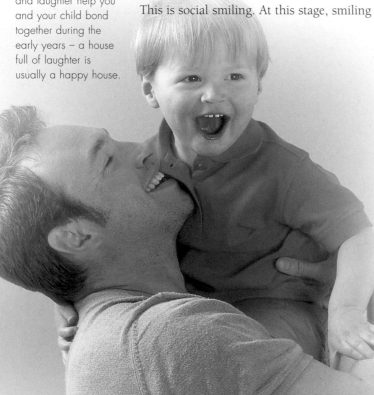

In the know... *Funny business*
Children are more attentive to stories read to them when the stories contain an element of humor – humor is an effective way to gain a child's interest and attention. Boys tend to recognize and respond to visual humor more easily than girls. When young boys and girls are shown cartoons, boys usually laugh sooner than girls.

becomes one of the ways in which infants explore their relationship with adults, learning what rewards they may gain by smiling, and coming to understand that their own smile rewards the adult, too.

Temperament

Smiling and laughter soon become characteristics that we describe as temperament. Some children laugh a lot, some are more serious. Laughter, or its absence, or crying become a spectrum of responses to new or different situations, and to people. They are used by your baby both to respond to others and to create responses in others; in other words, to test and explore relationships with people. Laughter, as well as crying, also may be used by infants and toddlers as a response to fear, so it does not always indicate happiness.

Body Language

As control of his upper limbs matures, your baby becomes able to make meaningful gestures with his arms. Holding his arms out toward you is a powerful way of attracting positive attention, and throwing objects away quickly becomes both a game and a way of indicating boredom or displeasure.

Children are particularly good at using their bodies to express aversion and negative emotions. Tantrums (see page 108) are good examples, but children also

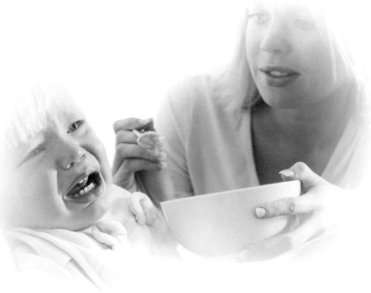

Expressing dislike
This mother is realizing her baby doesn't like his breakfast! Both his facial expression and posture indicate that at this moment he doesn't want to eat.

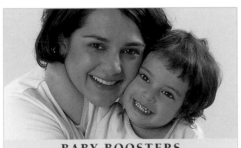

BABY BOOSTERS
LOVING, GENTLE TOUCH

Studies by psychologists reveal that in most families, the frequency of soft, warm physical contact between parent and baby diminishes after the first year. Toddlers are then able to stand on their own two feet and therefore are not so reliant on you to be carried everywhere or to be held during feeding, so that opportunities for loving, physical contact are often less. However, incidents of gentle touch between you and your toddler have greater emotional significance because they do not occur so often. That's why an unexpected hug, a surprising pat on his head, or an unpredictable arm around his shoulders will bring a warm smile to his face.

use facial expressions of disgust and gestures of rejection or refusal to emphasize feelings as a substitute for, or to accompany, verbal utterances or crying.

Imitation is body language that explicitly invites turn taking and interaction. It is commonly assumed that an infant imitates an adult, but when parents and infants are observed together, it is clear that the adult will sometimes be the one who imitates the baby's movement or behavior, thus encouraging the baby to imitate the adult in turn. Imitation quickly turns into reciprocal games such as peekaboo, and around the age of a year, children often start to mime: That is, use their hands in gestures that symbolize objects, such as holding imaginary phones to their ears, or substituting an object, such as a spoon, held to the ear like a phone. The phone symbol is especially interesting since it is often used to initiate a conversation with a parent or caregiver.

Another early body language is the farewell wave. Young children use this gesture not just to mean "good-bye," but also "I want to go now," or "I've had enough," or even "go away," according to context and how the child is feeling. This expressive gesture can convey far more than the child could manage verbally, and is thus a more sophisticated kind of language than words.

Tantrums

Perhaps the most powerful form of non-verbal communication your child displays during the preschool years is the tantrum – the unmistakable blend of body language in a tantrum tells you immediately he is frustrated and angry. A tantrum is usually triggered when your child's desires are blocked. For example, he wants to continue playing but you insist he stop because it is time for bed, or he wants another drink and you inform him that he has had enough. His temper can change and erupt in seconds.

Prevention is better than cure. Use your knowledge of his nonverbal communication to identify when a tantrum is developing, and then step in to calm him before he reaches boiling point. Watch out for the telltale signs that trouble is brewing. It might be that his face goes red, or that he starts to breathe heavily, or that he begins to whimper or whine – you'll be aware of the pretantrum gestures because you have seem them several times before. Once your early-warning system is alerted by his nonverbal behavior, do what you can to divert his energy and attention to something else.

In the know... Sign language

Babies can be taught expressive language skills as early as six to eight months, and around nine months can begin using signs to express basic needs. Some benefits of teaching your baby sign language are that by expressing ideas through the use of sign language, any potential frustration that can arise when he can't make himself understood may be reduced; the increased communication that comes from expressive language may strengthen the emotional bond between you and your baby, and your baby's use of sign language will often encourage communication.

However, it is important to emphasize spoken language as well. Your baby uses babbling sounds before he speaks. While encouraging him to use sign language it is still important that you pay attention to these early linguistic building blocks; pointing is easier for most babies to use than sign language, and research confirms that pointing improves attention as well as speech and language development. Sign language may interfere with the spontaneous growth in his use of spoken language, as, initially, he may learn to rely more on gestures than words.

Whether or not you teach your child sign language, the one-on-one time you spend communicating with him in any manner will benefit his language development.

speech

Your growing child's speech skills really lift off during the "Wonder Years." She transforms from a cooing and babbling baby into a confident and articulate child who is able to stand up in front of all her classmates and talk fluently about her recent family vacation.

This transformation is a combination of the inherent drive toward speech competence, which your child was born with, and the stimulation and encouragement you provide for her. No matter what age your child is, the more you talk to her, discuss with her, ask her questions, and listen to her stories, then the more likely she is to have good speech and language development. Bear in mind that after the babbling stage, your child's receptive language (the language that she understands) is always ahead of her expressive language (the words she is able to say), which means she understands much more than she can put into words.

The stages in acquiring speech

* **Around 12–15 months:** Your child may be able to use up to three or four clear words, although some children don't reach this stage until months later. She will also be able to follow basic directions. Hearing is usually sharp at this age.

* **Around 18–24 months:** She uses around 50 different words, either singly or combined into two-words phrases. Most words are nouns, referring to specific familiar objects or to people whom she knows well (e.g. her siblings, her pet dog, her friend).

* **At 2–3 years:** Vocabulary is almost 200 words now, and although mainly still nouns, many of them are general rather than specific (e.g. "car," "doll"). She also uses pronouns. However, she still makes minor errors such as "tat" for "cat."

* **At 3–4 years:** She uses upwards of 1,000 different words, and understands a lot more than this. Sentences are longer, containing many verbs and adjectives. Most of the earlier "baby" mannerisms have been dropped. She asks questions.

* **At 4–5 years:** Your child has a spoken vocabulary of approximately 1,500 words. Her speech begins to resemble adult speech in the way it communicates her feelings and ideas. She uses the past tense and other word endings. Your child should speak clearly enough so that an observer who is listening closely can understand most of what she says.

Simple speech

Simple speech is the stage of development when a child not only says her first words, but is able to string two or three words together to make a phrase, and there is a very wide range of ages over which it develops. For instance, while around half of all infants have achieved their first words by the age of 12 months, and most

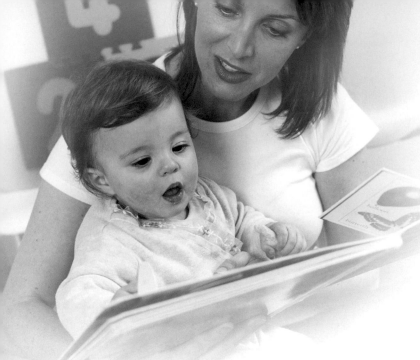

Books are fun
"Reading" a picture book with you gives your child exposure to the words for objects outside her immediate experience, and nourishes not just her language, but her imagination as well. By reading books with you, as well as having her concentration and attention span rewarded, your child begins to associate words, language, and imagination with an emotionally pleasant and fun experience.

have attained this by the age of 15 months, there are many children who do not make real progress in language until well past their second birthday. In general, how well your child understands is a better indicator of language development than her actual spoken words. Talk to your pediatrician if you are concerned about speech delay, but in some cases all your child needs is more time for her speech to develop. Often these children are referred for speech therapy, they then go on to make normal progress and quickly catch up with their peers. In some cases "delayed" speech runs in the family.

Emerging from babbling, the first sounds that become words to which meaning is definitely attached are usually "mama" and "dada" in English-speaking countries. Following close behind, and depending on local culture and the words to which they are exposed, come greetings like "hi" or "hiya," farewells like "bye," and names used for brothers, sisters, close friends or relatives, or a family pet. The

emergence of these words is usually highly rewarded by the attention of parents and other family members, so the reinforcement for the child is very strong.

Initially, when your baby wants something, she uses the "point and shout" method, but as she learns to use words, she can substitute language for important objects, and these words tend to come very soon after words like "mama" and "dada." First the word itself is used, and the loudness with which it is used conveys urgency. Then a word may be coupled with another to make the utterance more specific, like "hi Dada." Strikingly, words with two different syllables (like "doggie") emerge very soon after both words with one syllable (dog), and the same syllables repeated (mama, dada). It's usually only a short step to combining different words, and to the child, there is no difference between one two-syllable word and two one-syllable words.

The way in which words are acquired varies a lot between children. For instance, some expand their initial number of words very quickly, but acquire mostly the words for objects and persons (nouns). Others acquire words more slowly but balance the kinds of words they learn: They learn not just nouns, but description words (adjectives), action words (verbs), and others. The main use of language when speech is at its simplest is to express needs and wants, usually by using the name of the object that is required ("teddy bear").

The richness of a child's environment is a powerful driver for learning new words and language. This is not just about hearing words, it is about hearing them as part of an interaction with other people. It is about the reinforcement and rewards that the child gets in relation to language, and it is about exposure to words in context.

Increasing vocabulary

Most children's vocabularies increase dramatically in the months following their first words. You'll soon lose count of the new words your child picks up. However, the way that words are acquired varies between children. According to their personality, children seem to have preferences for some words over others.

Since children do not all acquire the same kinds of words as each other, it should not be surprising that the use of language varies between children, too. Some children are "expressers" who use language primarily to express their needs and feelings, while others, sometimes called "referrers," use their language mostly to identify objects and people. These traits are often apparent from a very early stage of language use.

As the first words expand into a larger vocabulary, the use of words for classes of object changes, too. An example is "doggie," which may initially be used by a child as the word for any furry, four-legged creature, but the word then becomes specific to "dogs" as new words are gained that allow the child to specify, for instance, cat, horse, and cow. There is then no need to call all of them "doggie."

Aiding your child's progress

The words that children hear are the words they learn. Your role in providing these words is hugely important for your child. Typically, the child of a quiet caregiver will simply not pick up words as fast as one who has a caregiver who constantly talks with her child. Yet most of the time, very young children do not imitate or mimic sounds and words from parents or caregivers. What seems to be important is that parents engage with their child, making conversation, and try to understand their child's first attempts at words even though they are sometimes almost impossible to get. Listening to a child's words, and saying them back, seems to be the key. Children sometimes struggle with particular sounds and need encouragement and reward to get them right. Repeating words, and using actions or pictures to accompany them, all help young children to get both new words and new meanings.

Reading to young children, even using the most basic board books, is good for encouraging them to try new words, as well as providing a time of close attention and emotional warmth. Some children respond best to familiar books, while others seem to prefer new ones. It doesn't matter what you read or if you use words that aren't even on the pages. "Reading" together enables children to relate words to others, and to learn that altering the endings of words can change meaning: For example, plurals such as dog to dogs, cow to cows. Then they try mouse to "mouses" and quickly find out that the "rules" of language get broken, but only on certain occasions. They learn that changing the order of words can also create new meanings, like the difference between "It is a cat" and "Is it a cat?".

Building a vocabulary and learning the rules of the language go hand-in-hand.

Similarly, language and vocabulary join together to form conversation. Conversation is partly about taking turns, but it also allows children to experiment not just with new words, but also with ways of saying them, and ways of joining words together to create new meanings. Conversation is also about listening, so you have the opportunity to demonstrate to your child the importance of listening, and to reward that behavior in your child. With both children and parents, some are much better at listening than others. Good listening skills, and plenty of opportunity to practice, are both important in helping your young child to build up her vocabulary.

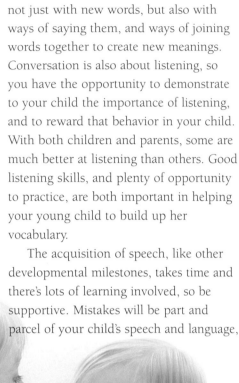

The acquisition of speech, like other developmental milestones, takes time and there's lots of learning involved, so be supportive. Mistakes will be part and parcel of your child's speech and language, so don't make it a big deal when these natural errors occur. Try to listen when your child wants to talk. Even though you may be busy with other things, set aside time to have a discussion. Toddlers, especially, often are unsure of the exact words to use or maybe can't talk well enough so that they need time to speak. When your child speaks to you, don't rush her, but do help her stay on track. A four-year-old, for example, can easily lose the point of a discussion if she isn't given a gentle reminder from you.

Look at your child and make eye contact when you talk to her; this helps her focus attention on your comments. And encourage her to look at you. Remind her, as she gets older, to make eye contact when speaking to another person. The social actions accompanying speech will be increasingly important.

Help your child expand her vocabulary by telling her the names of different objects, and asking her questions about things she is doing – like what is she drawing, for example. Use as much detail as possible. Instead of saying "put your toys away" say "please put your toys in the closet." Also, tell her the meanings of words. You may find her questions about word meanings irritating, but this helps her extend her vocabulary further.

From the time your child is a toddler, use your normal speaking style, but try to speak more slowly, using less complex sentence structures so that she can tune in more easily. Always provide a good model of language. For example, if your child says "Daddy car," you can reply by saying "Yes, that's right, Dad's car is outside."

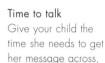

Time to talk
Give your child the time she needs to get her message across, even if she uses only sounds or gestures.

understanding begins

Infants and young children have an ability to understand language, and hence commands, that runs far ahead of their ability to express things all the way through their preschool years. Even very young babies understand the tone of voice, and therefore the emotional content, if not the words themselves. Young babies pick up emotional cues, and may become distressed if they sense distress or anxiety in an adult; on the other hand, they are easily comforted by hearing soothing or reassuring sounds.

How understanding develops

* *Up to 8 months:* Although the connection between tone of voice and emotion is far in advance of an understanding of language, your infant may appear to have some linguistic understanding a few weeks before he utters his first meaningful words.

* *Around 8–9 months:* Your child's ability to follow instructions starts around now; he may be able to do what you ask as long as it involves a simple physical hand movement that he can see and it requires him to interact with you. For instance, he may try to hand you a toy he is holding if you ask him for it in a playful way while holding out your hand.

* *Around 13–14 months:* Your toddler begins to understand basic instructions that are not tied to an object immediately in front of him. He knows, for instance, what you mean when you tell him "No, you can't have any more" – his probable tantrum that immediately follows is proof that he definitely knows what you mean.

* *By 18 months:* Your toddler is beginning to be able to follow a simple command that contains one piece of information such as "Please put the ball in the box."

* *From 3 years:* Your child should be able to process and complete more complex commands involving at least two pieces of information due to increases in his thinking skills and memory, for instance, "Please bring me the book and put the doll in your room."

* *From 4 years:* Your child starts to ask questions, though it's not until he is about five years of age that he can think carefully about the questions he would like to ask.

Providing explanations

Most of the commands you give your child will be nonnegotiable, and you will expect him to carry them out. But at times your child won't want to do what you ask, perhaps because he is busy with another activity or because he thinks your instructions are uninteresting or unimportant. That's why it helps to give him an explanation. Point out to your child that you want him to stop playing with the game because it's time to go shopping and you'd like him to get ready. Start giving this type of explanation from the toddler stage onward

– he won't fully understand the reasons, but it will encourage him to think beyond his own immediate wishes. Explanations help your child realize why you are asking him to behave in a particular way.

In addition, point out the emotional consequences of his following your instructions. For instance, you could tell him that you'll feel good if he puts his clothes back in the closet, or that his brother will be sad if he doesn't take care of his toys. Linking the instruction to an emotional outcome in this way makes your instruction more significant for your child, and he is therefore more likely to respond positively to it.

Asking questions

Questions are a great way for a child to start a conversation. They also arise from his natural curiosity about his environment, and the things that go on in it. For the young child, the desire to learn about the world is not in any sense a luxury, it is a necessity. And as all parents come to realize, it is a lot easier for a child to ask a question than for the parent to provide a good answer. Sometimes questions are asked to which there is no answer, or sometimes the answer simply can't be properly understood by a young child. Yet even very young children need to be taken seriously, and even the hardest questions need some kind of answer. Answer your child's questions as best you can but you can also tell him that there are some questions that don't have easy answers (e.g. "What happens when you die?"). In such cases it is fine to answer

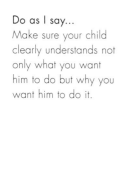

Do as I say...
Make sure your child clearly understands not only what you want him to do but why you want him to do it.

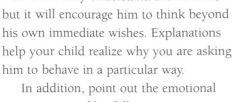
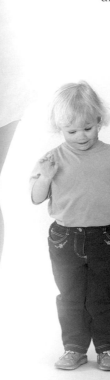
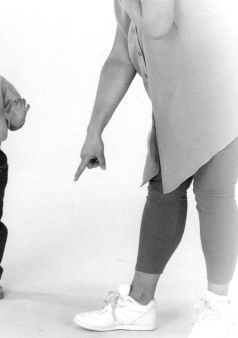

simply and provide only the information that is appropriate for your child at his current age.

The ability to ask questions comes from being able to make complex sentences, as well as to think in abstract terms. Questions may arise because a child has not been successful in solving some challenge presented by things happening around him: he may not understand these events, and needs more information to make sense of things.

From about four years of age, children start to ask questions; this is when they usually have enough language, and sufficient intellectual skill, to frame a question. Somewhere between four and six years old is often the peak time for constantly asking questions, and five year olds may start to think through both the kind of problem they are trying to solve, and the kinds of question they want to ask, before putting it into words. But even before then, children typically think about choices, weigh up the possibilities, and ask questions about them. For instance, offered the chance to go to the store with Dad, or stay at home with Mom, there may be a question about whether Dad might buy a treat, or whether Mom will play a game. The answer to the question might determine whether store or home looks like the better choice. The child is considering the future possibilities for each scenario, and imagining how each might feel, before deciding whether to go or stay. This requires a fairly high level of abstract thought.

Questions come in all sizes. Big ones might relate to birth and death ("Where do babies come from?" Or on the death of a pet "Where did he go to?"). Others may be "What if…?" type questions ("What if the store is closed?"), and others may start "Why…?", as in connection with behavior ("Why did you shout at Annie?"), or about events ("Why does it rain?") It is important not to deter children from asking, and just as important to try to answer with honesty, even if all you have to say is "I don't know."

Aiding your child's progress

You can help your child to develop both his thinking and style of questioning by asking "What if…?" and "How does" questions of your child. This helps your child to develop different styles of interaction as well as to explore the world in an abstract way. Adults generally try to encourage children to ask about the way something works, rather than allow the child to break it open to try to find out.

In terms of expanding your child's thinking, it is often better to ask open-ended questions like "Why do you like your friend?", which are more challenging than closed questions such as "Do you like your friend?", which have yes or no answers. For instance, on setting out for the post office, you might say "What shall we do if the post office is closed?" – and there could be all sorts of answers to that open question. On the other hand, if you just say "If the post office is closed, shall we come straight home?" – the answer is most likely "yes" or "no." Other possibilities may exist, but your child is clearly not being encouraged to suggest them when the question is closed.

food for thought

Good nutrition, along with regular physical activity, is essential for your child to develop his full potential. To make it easier for parents to ensure their children "eat right," scientists have updated the concept of the food pyramid, which is an easy way to visualize the nutritional needs for children two years old and up. The most up-to-date version consists of six categories that should be eaten every day, though the amounts of each differs. For more information visit www.mypyramid.gov.

Grains

This, the largest food group, consists of wheat, rice, barley, oats, rye, millet, and quinoa, and the breads, cereals, and pasta made from them. Whole grains are rich in vitamins and minerals and these should be chosen over more refined products, even if they are fortified with nutrients. Grains provide children with complex carbohydrates that are essential for sustained energy and for regulating blood sugar levels. Fluctuating blood sugar levels lead to poor concentration and memory and children are particularly susceptible. Half of the grain servings should be whole grain products.

In the know... *Breastfeeding*
The American Academy of Pediatrics and many other experts encourage women to breastfeed as long as possible, one year or even longer, because breastmilk provides optimal nutrition and protection against infections.

Vegetables

Filled with essential nutrients such as a wide range of vitamins and minerals, vegetables must make a major contribution to the daily diet. Because differently colored vegetables (i.e. green vegetables like broccoli and spinach or orange ones like carrots and sweet potatoes) contain different nutrients, your child should be offered a variety.

Milk

Vital for building strong bones, the calcium found in milk, and dairy foods such as yogurt and cheese, also has positive effects on the brain as it is important for nerve and hormone function. Children need two cups every day from this food group.

Fruit

Like vegetables, this food group is also filled with essential vitamins and minerals. Again, as with vegetables, different colored fruit provide different nutrients, so make certain you feed your child a variety. Fruit juice should be limited to no more than 4–6 ounces per day of 100 percent fruit juice with no added sugar.

Meat and beans

This protein-rich group is made up of lean or low-fat beef, lamb, and pork; chicken, turkey, and eggs; fish; nuts, seeds, lentils, peas, and beans. Protein foods contain amino acids, which are necessary to make key brain chemicals. Red meat is particularly rich in iron, which is necessary to keep all the body's tissues and organs functioning well.

It is recommended that young children only eat fish and shellfish that are low in mercury, such as shrimp, canned light tuna, salmon, pollock, and catfish. Nuts and seeds should be avoided until four years of age since they are highly allergenic and a potential choking hazard. If there's a family history of food allergies, hold off on introducing fish, shellfish, nuts, or seeds to your child's diet until you talk to your pediatrician first.

Oils

Part of the food pyramid, though not a food group, a small amount of oil is needed on a daily basis to keep the nervous system functioning well. As well as liquid cooking oils such as corn oil, soybean oil, and canola oil, beneficial oils can be found in fish and nuts.

Water

One of the most important things you can do for your child's health is to get her used to drinking water at a young age. Water is important to keep your child's body healthy and working properly.

Cancel the caffeine

Caffeine is a stimulant found in certain products – many of which children like, such as soft drinks, chocolate, and frozen yogurt. Eating or drinking such items can have many negative effects on your child's health, including causing jitteriness, difficulty concentrating, sleeplessness, headaches, dental problems, obesity and dehydration.

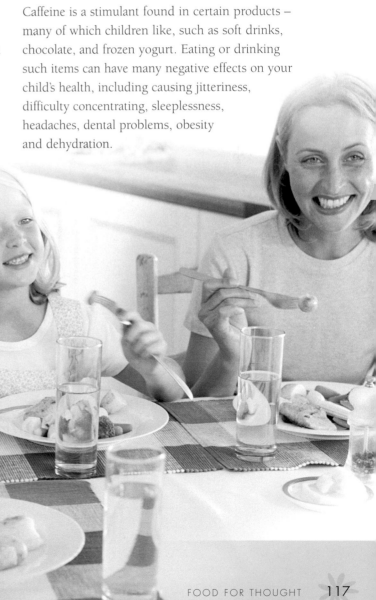

mastering increasingly complex activities

More complex activities develop with the increased intellectual abilities that come with age. To do complex things requires memory, planning, skills to carry out tasks, and learning from the whole process. All of these develop rapidly from your child's second year onward.

Trial and error as a general plan for exploring things becomes much more sophisticated by the age of two, and the amount of persistence that your child is prepared to put in to trying to understand objects and make them work increases greatly. So most activities, even though they may still be quite simple, commonly last much longer than when he was younger.

Now is the time, too, when activities start to sort themselves into different domains: there are things to be done with crayons and paper, with toys, and reading.

Dressing, washing, cleaning teeth, brushing hair, and eating – all these can now be done better and faster. Your child will have learned that washing and dressing consist of certain smaller tasks that need to be done more or less in the right order if the whole process is to work out – for instance, socks have to go on before shoes. Your assistance may be refused sometimes, even if it would speed up the process, and you may find your child will often make a running commentary on what he is doing.

As your child gains greater height and physical strength, he also becomes more

dexterous, and this means he can engage in outdoor play which is more complicated and sustained, whether it is using playground equipment or exploring different habitats such as the beach and park. Another type of more complex play involves imaginative role-playing. This may involve putting a doll to bed or nursing a sick teddy bear.

Once your child is around three, he'll have the ability to stick with an activity for longer; this is a prerequisite to functioning in a more complex way than before, and this means becoming less distracted by external events and more able to focus on the task in hand, even if it is a bit difficult.

Also, if he gets stuck, your child will be more able to frame a question that will help him to deal with the problem and to come up with different solutions – for instance, when playing with a simple construction toy where different-sized bricks can be fashioned into structures, to choose the appropriate pieces.

Activities such as conversation with older people – child care teachers or older relatives – take on new dimensions because your child has so much more language to use, and more complicated stories to tell. At the same time, his play becomes more imaginative and complicated; he may act out roles such as being Mommy or Daddy, or set up complicated scenarios with model animals.

Without overwhelming him, or presenting impossibly complicated tasks, you can help your child to play in an increasingly sophisticated and complex way. But even just left to himself, your child will find ways to stretch himself and to invent imaginative new ways to entertain himself.

Curiosity

Your child is a natural learner. He instinctively tries to make sense of everything he sees, hears, and touches. This natural curiosity – his desire to discover the undiscovered – drives him to learn more at every opportunity. As a baby, he looks at, touches, smells, and chews anything he can get his hands on. Everything he sees represents a new and exciting opportunity to explore and learn more. And this intrinsic motivation to reach new heights continues to drive him throughout childhood.

As an active toddler, you need to keep a close eye on him because he likes to search every cupboard, open every box, and empty out every container. He's not purposely being bad, he just wants to find out how things work.

By the time he reaches school age, his curiosity is channeled and more controlled, and the new learning opportunities involving reading and counting are the means to satisfy his eagerness to acquire more knowledge.

Promoting early educational skills

Your child's thirst for learning means that he may show an interest in reading and numbers before he actually starts school. Let your child's interest and ability guide you. If he seems ready, you can help teach him letters and numbers before he starts school.

There is a lot of reading and counting that can occur naturally throughout your child's daily routine. For instance, he will start to recognize the names of stores that he frequently visits with you. Likewise, he may start to count out his grapes before eating them. Praise him when he demonstrates these early learning skills – he thrives under your approval. You'll find that the sort of information he acquires through his natural thirst for learning will give him a good start to formal schooling.

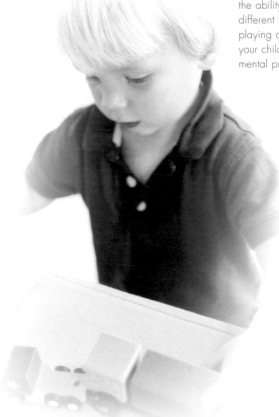

Master of the game
Greater concentration and "stick-to-itivity" and the ability to separate different kinds of playing demonstrate your child's mature mental process.

self-perception

Throughout childhood the way your child perceives herself changes. During toddlerhood, your child has more sense of herself as an individual but assumes that you see the world as she sees it. By the time she is five or six years old, however, your child can describe herself reasonably accurately; has a sense of who she is, and how she relates to the people around her.

Personal intelligence includes the ability to think about and distinguish between feelings, recognize them as discrete emotions, and then use them to direct behavior. This intelligence is one of your child's greatest keys to success in life. It will not only help her understand what she is good at (and bad), but it will help her set realistic goals when she is older.

Shock to the system
The arrival of a sibling can challenge a child's perception of herself, as her place in the family is no longer what it was.

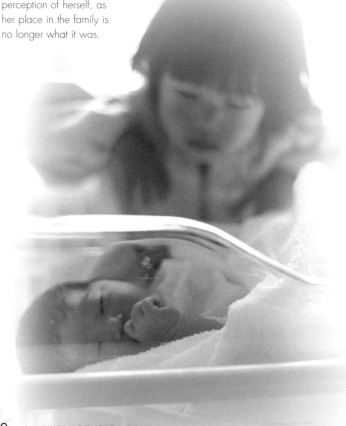

I am me
One of the early signs that your baby knows she is a separate individual is when she starts to make decisions about her own behavior. Smiling is a good example. When your baby gives you a big grin in response to your smile, this proves that she is aware you and she are separate, that she can process the sensory information, which tells her you are smiling, and that she is able to decide to reply to with a beaming facial expression of her own.

Realizing that she has control over her body is an essential stage in developing her perception of who she is, and research suggests this understanding emerges as early as three months.

How self-perception develops
From birth on, your baby will become aware that she is able to make things happen, that what she does has an influence on others. This is referred to as "personal agency" and it develops gradually along the following lines:
* *Newborn:* It doesn't take your baby long to forge a link in her mind between her crying loudly and your appearance in front of her. Within a few weeks, she learns that crying is an effective strategy for bringing you to her.

* **Around 3–6 months:** With increasing hand-control, she is able to hold a rattle in her hands, move it vigorously, and cause it to make a noise. She delights in the knowledge that she has this control over the object.

* **Around 6–9 months:** While sitting up without support, she is able to think that she wants a particular toy, and then reach for it. Her ability to match together her perception, desire, and control in one action boosts her enjoyment.

* **Around 1 year:** Your toddler's developing thinking skills allow her to plan more complex cause-and-effect operations. For instance, if she sees her toy resting out of reach on a towel, she pulls the towel toward herself to get the toy.

* **Around 2–3 years:** Her self-perception is so strong that it pushes aside consideration of others. Many tantrums occur at this age because your child refuses to accept that what you want is more important than what she wants.

* **Around 3–4 years:** She knows a lot more about herself now, for instance, whether she is a girl or a boy, her name and age. She can list these traits for you, when asked.

Dealing with emotions

Recognizing emotions both in herself and others will enable your child to express them and to understand why she and others feel the way they do. This can help her to deal with difficult situations and to react more appropriately and effectively as she gets older. Instead of flying into a tantrum when some treat is refused, she may be able to "negotiate" a more favorable settlement if she learns to keep her emotions in check.

With your young baby, she either has times when she is crying or not crying. Gradually she acquires a range of sounds that reflect her happiness or unhappiness. During your baby's second year, she will begin to more clearly express distinct emotions. Perhaps the most obvious is the pride she takes in her achievements, which doesn't stop her from looking to you for constant positive reinforcement as she crawls, stands up, and eventually walks, among other achievements.

Soon you will notice more subtle responses as she will be able to express shades of amusement, and degrees of anger and frustration.

- - - - - - - - - - - - - - - - - - - -

In the know... My name is...

Another sign of your infant's growing sense of self-perception is her recognition that her name actually refers to herself. In the early weeks and months, her name is used constantly when people talk to her, play with her, or hug her. But that doesn't mean she knows the word designates her, as opposed to any other person or object. Your child's genuine understanding that her name indicates her and no one else does not usually emerge until between the ages of 12 and 15 months.

- - - - - - - - - - - - - - - - - - - -

game play

The tiny word "play" doesn't do justice either to its importance to babies, young children, and throughout life, or to its fundamental place in learning and development. Play is many related things: Exploring, satisfying curiosity, testing, probing, experimenting, influencing, and fun! It is spontaneous and meaningful to your child. When it involves responses and rewards involving others, it becomes a game or a series of games.

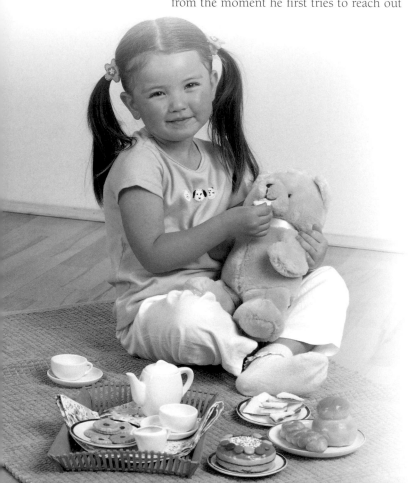

Make believe
Children use play to experiment with feelings as well as to exercise their imaginations.

Play is the dominant activity that children do in their waking hours. It is the foundation for competition and collaboration, for learning, abstraction, and reasoning. It leads to who we are, how we behave, how we think, and what we do.

Your child learns through play, right from the moment he first tries to reach out to touch the rattle dangled in front of him. Play is the means through which he engages with the world, whether it is creative play (using art and craft materials), exploratory play (as he investigates the cupboard), physical play (when he rolls, crawls, walks, or climbs), or imaginative play (when he pretends to be someone else).

Early play
Toys and other playthings become important around six months of age. Purpose-made toys are never strictly essential to learning, as children will invent their own games and toys anyway, but well-designed toys can provide stimuli for exploring and discovering new things. On the other hand, safe, common household items such as large wooden spoons and saucepan lids can provide hours of fun. Blocks, soft toys, and board books are good choices as they can be manipulated and interacted with.

Your young baby should have toys that stimulate all his senses. They should be of different textures, colors, and shapes, and make interesting noises – especially when he holds or shakes them.

Your toddler will enjoy putting in and taking out games involving containers, stacking toys, and shape sorters but his main task is about discovering the world using his newfound height and mobility.

Your toddler will rely on simple, physical, and usually nonverbal means to do things. He will explore simple objects in a physical way; for instance, he may try to push a toy car through a gap that is too small, and he will "test" new objects for whether they have wheels, whether they can fit in a box, and what they taste like.

When he's a little older, and he has acquired the skill of wrist rotation, he'll enjoy unscrewing and opening things and will engage in imaginative play such as dressing up or in drawing, painting, and modeling.

Game playing

While much of your child's play in the early years does not involve anyone else – toddler play is commonly solitary, parallel with another child, or done with an adult – part of his play experience centers around games. In contrast to other forms of play, most games involve interaction with at least one other person. Through games, your child develops new skills, learns new social rules, and enhances his understanding. There are so many benefits to this form of play – and games are good fun, too!

Games begin very early in life. The interactions and communication that are first established between a parent and baby are themselves a form of game play. Very early on, your baby is exploring behaviors and noises for their effects on you or another caregiver, and this is a particular

kind of exploratory, experimental play. Your baby is trying to find out what works to get his parent's attention – he is "asking" himself, "How many smiles must I make? What noises?" Just as playing with sounds becomes the foundation for language, through gaming with his parents' responses and emotions, your child learns about relationships.

A genuine game involves the following components. First, awareness of the other person's response – it wouldn't be a game if your infant didn't react to your behavior. Your baby does this instinctively. For instance, when you smile at him and tickle him, he giggles in response – his behavior is affected by what he sees and feels you do. He is too young to make an action himself as part of the game, but he will be able to do that eventually.

Most games require one person to behave in a certain way while the others wait for their turns. Because this turn taking requires patience and an awareness of the game's structure, it may not be until around the age of two or three years that your child can manage this without tears. Before that stage of maturity, he may lose interest or burst out crying when he realizes someone else is ahead of him.

Finally, every game has rules – peekaboo has simple rules (he lies there while you hide your face behind your hands and make it reappear suddenly) whereas bingo is more complex. Your child probably won't able to participate fully in a game with rules until he is around the age of four or five.

Stages in game play

❋ *Until about 18 months:* Your toddler will have little interest in games that involve him interacting with his peers. He is happy with his own company, and he does not pay much attention to other children playing around him. He concentrates only on what he is playing with, ignoring the rest.

❋ *Between 18 months and 3 years:* Your child plays alongside others his age but they all still play independently and don't interact in games. He watches what they do with curiosity and he might even move over to sit beside them, without actually joining in their games.

❋ *From 3 years:* Your child may now be ready to fully participate in games with his pals. He may actually play together with others, share ideas and toys, listen to another's suggestions, and modify his own actions to merge with theirs.

❋ *4–5 years:* Your child has a strong need for playing games with his peers. Games allow him to become part of the social group.

Games and learning

Your child learns a great deal from playing games with his friends or siblings. It's not just that he learns the rules of the game – although that does improve his understanding, memory, and thinking skills – it's that he also develops awareness of other people's feelings. He learns about

Playing with others
This is a vital stage in your child's development as it's never too early to learn from one's peers.

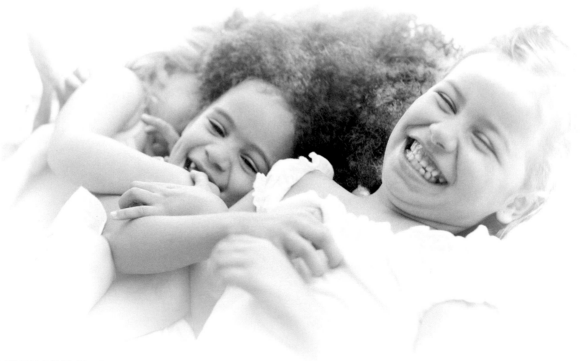

reciprocity. When he played on his own, he made all the choices. In games, however, your child has to get along well with the others or the game cannot take place. That's why playing games with others his own age enhances your child's social relationships and encourages his sensitivity.

Learning occurs in other ways during games with his peers. First, your child learns directly. For example, when it is his turn to pick up the dice and roll it, he learns about the shape and feel of the dice, the sound it makes when it leaves his hand, and the way he has to throw hard enough for it to roll but not so hard that it rolls off the board.

Then there is incidental learning. While playing a game, he learns along the way; for instance, he learns that all pieces for the game fit into the box and that the counters can be stacked neatly into a pile.

Third, your child learns instrumentally. This occurs when all the children playing a game together face a common problem, which they have to solve in order to progress. For instance, they realize that in order to play a game of catch they have to find where the equipment is kept.

PARENTAL PARTICIPATION

To help your child to learn, it's important to create the right environment.

Provide your child with the "right" toys

These are things that are safe and interesting without being overwhelming and with which he can engage actively. They also should include things your child can operate himself without extra help, such as dolls, balls, and blocks. Try to understand what engages your child and provide him with those activities. He may prefer puzzles to drawing, for example.

Vary your child's environment

Rotate the toys offered to your child – always remembering to put away any that he doesn't play with or maybe has outgrown or has damaged. Teach him the value of giving away or donating toys that he has outgrown. Read stories to him every day and try to engage him in new activities.

Include yourself in games

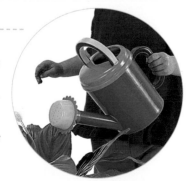

Your child will learn more from you than objects so make sure you make him part of your activities, even if it doesn't seem like play. On the other hand, avoid temptation to be overly directive; give him the space to play the way he wants.

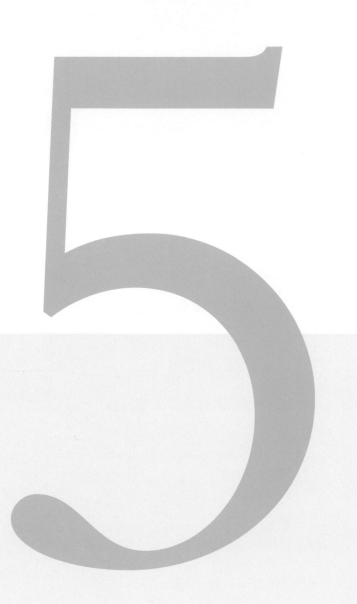
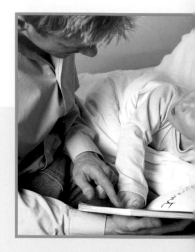

social and emotional development

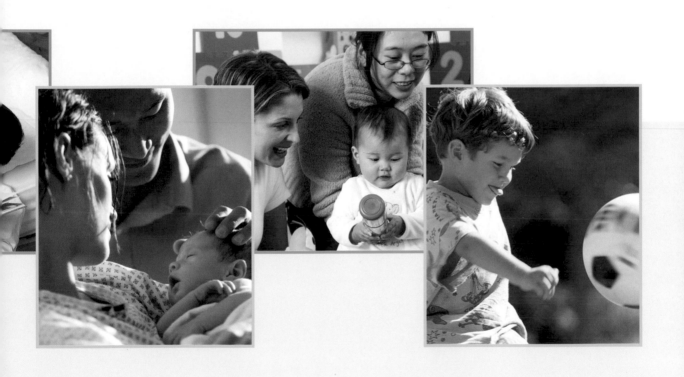

understanding the stages

First-time parents are often surprised that their baby seems to have a strong personality early in life. They may be even more surprised when a second child arrives with a personality different from the first. Research shows that distinctive personality characteristics are discernible in babies as young as three months old. Sociability is part of personality and, like other personality traits, is particularly influenced by genetics.

There is no doubt that your child is an individual from an early age. She will find her own ways of showing you how she feels, as well as her likes and dislikes. Your baby will start to communicate with you from birth.

Crying is the first means she uses but from about two weeks of age, she will start to make other little noises. Soon she will make noises in response to what you are saying. At around six weeks she will smile at you, too. If you hold your face about eight inches away from hers, she will watch your lips moving and will soon start to move her own in a similar way.

As early as three months of age, she will anticipate what is to come and smile excitedly as you prepare for her favorite activities; at about four months she will turn away from things she does not want.

Babies are very sociable creatures, who enjoy the company both of adults and children. Your baby will soon learn to chat to you in her own way and will love playing with you. There are lots of fun things you and your baby can do together.

The sequence of events

In just one year your child will change from a tiny baby to a robust toddler who will be affectionate and will show her independence, perhaps by trying to feed herself with a spoon or by helping you to get her dressed.

As she becomes more alert and her senses develop, your baby will become more aware of those around her. Initially, she will be outgoing and friendly, pleased to meet new people as well as to see those

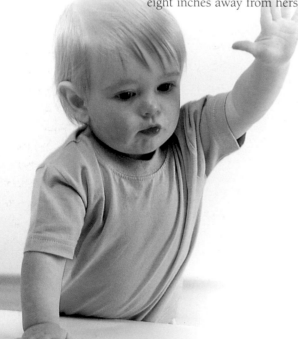

Bye-bye
Babies of around a year will wave good-bye when you leave them.

she knows well. However, over the coming months, she will start to become wary of strangers, looking to you for comfort and reassurance when meeting someone new.

Once your baby begins to walk, she will happily toddle and later run toward you. She will soon learn to run away from you, too! This newfound mobility also will enable her to take her first major steps toward independence, although she will have been trying to do some things for herself already.

You can watch your child's sociability and personality develop as you do her movement and other skills. Every child goes through an independence-seeking phase. That behavior occurs at the same time as a parent is trying to set limits for appropriate behaviors. The result – tantrums. At this age, toddlers have the will to do many things but cannot always follow their desires, whether this is due to limitations in their own skills or limits imposed by their parents. Whatever the reasons, two year olds often express their frustrations and anger through aggressive behavior (see page 145).

All children go through the "terrible two's," but some start earlier than age two and some start later. Eventually, this behavior will resolve and parents will find their children become more amenable and willing to follow instructions.

Over the coming years, children continue to test boundaries and try to assert their independence, but at the same time, parents can start to reason with them and may be able to explain another's point of view. This will not always work, however. Young children often want to make their own choices – you may long

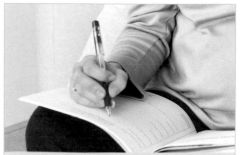

BABY BOOSTERS
KEEPING RECORDS

Social development is monitored along with movement, hearing, and vision. Your observations and experiences with your child will form a major part of any assessments made. It is worth keeping a note of your baby's milestones and when they are achieved – like the first time she smiles in response to you. At the time, you think you will never forget her achievements but later you probably won't remember exactly at what age they occurred. This will especially be the case if you have more children. As well as being a reminder for you and your partner, this record will also be invaluable if your baby ever requires further assessment.

for the days when your child was happy to put on what was laid out for her in the morning rather than choosing her own mismatched selection of clothes!

Sharing is another issue with which young children need time to come to terms; not only do they need to learn to share their possessions but also to share their parents with siblings and others.

Throughout the "Wonder Years," you will see your child achieve certain milestones at or around particular ages,

Signs of sociability and the emergence of personality occur at approximately these ages.

1 month: Becomes more alert and responsive.
Will stop crying when picked up and talked to.
Will soon learn to recognize your face, voice, and smell.

5–6 weeks: Makes first smile responsively.
Starts to make noises to express feelings of contentment or unhappiness.

2 months: Shows pleasure in recognizing parent by smiling, punching the air with the arms, or kicking the legs.
Has longer wakeful periods and starts to take an interest in what is going on.
Will respond with noises when talked to.

3 months: Will look up when being fed.
Starts to anticipate enjoyable things – will get excited when sees bottle being prepared and probably at bath time.
Loves being with parent, happy to see siblings and other relatives, and likely to be outgoing and to enjoy meeting new people.

4 months: Starts to express dislikes by turning away from unwanted things.
Beginning to develop a variety of facial expressions as well as smiles to express feelings.

5 months: Will look at face in the mirror but doesn't know who it is.
May start to babble to express happiness or unhappiness.
Will be very affectionate – pats parent and gets excited when he or she is seen approaching; may get upset when parent walks away.

6 months: Will love playing with parents.
First signs of stranger awareness may show.

7–8 months: Is more aware of strangers now; looks at them seriously rather than with open smile.

9 months: Starts to make very clear likes and dislikes; may stiffen body and resist doing certain things but will eagerly do others.
Will communicate with you through a variety of noises, both happy and unhappy.

10 months: Starts to communicate with gestures.
Holds arms out to be picked up.
Stranger awareness is obvious.

12 months: Shows early signs of independence; may drink out of a cup and self-feed with fingers.

15 months: Very loving and affectionate, may like parents around for reassurance and encouragement.
May carry a "security" object.
Starts to be helpful; may assist with dressing.

15–18 months: Will self-feed with a spoon.
May become frustrated when unable to do what is wanted; tantrums often begin about now.

18 months:	Shows more signs of independence and may be able to play alone for short periods.
	Will love to help with household tasks.
2 years:	More able to do things alone; for example, may be able to put shoes on.
	"Let's pretend" becomes a more prominent feature of play.
	Plays alongside another but not together.
	Is not prepared to share; clings to toys if someone else wants them.
2–3 years:	Starts to play with another a little.
3 years:	Tantrums have often settled by now.
	Is likely to be happier to follow your instructions.
4 years:	Sharing begins; more understanding about taking turns.
	Signs of independence more evident.
	Frequent quarrels may erupt between strong-willed friends.
	Has preferred friends and will be affectionate toward them.
	May demonstrate a sense of humor.
	More patient and a little more able to wait for things.
5 years:	Seems more grown-up.
	Shows empathy for others.
	Concerned about siblings and often takes care of them.

but at the same time, her character will shine through. By the age of five, you will feel you know her well. By then she will be more independent and at the same time will show more concern for those around her. She will also understand that other people have feelings and needs, too.

Aiding your child's progress

All children need a loving, nurturing environment in which they can thrive and develop. The way parents react to their achievements and their disappointments will help to shape their personalities for the years ahead.

It is very important to remain positive as much as possible, to respond to your child's needs quickly, and to take an interest in all that she does. But at the same time, you need to set boundaries for

Let's pretend
Make-believe play, which often mimics adult behavior, begins at around the age of two and continues for many years.

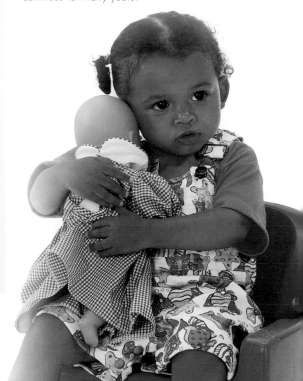

your child so that she comes to understand the difference between right and wrong.

It is very important never to say a child has a certain type of personality, for example "shy" or "bossy." She should be allowed to develop her personality and social skills unimpeded by the views or expectations of others. It is particularly important to avoid talking to other people about your child's personality or behavior in front of her. Even young children can pick up the meaning of a conversation without understanding every word. Be accepting – although you may be a very confident person, your child may be less outgoing. It is important not to impose your own social behavior on your child, but to encourage her to be herself and to make friends and socialize in her own way.

Another key part of being a parent is setting the right example – your child will spend more time with you than with anyone else. You need to show her the correct way to play and interact with others by being polite, sharing things with her, and showing her how to take turns.

Parallel play
Each of these toddlers is involved with playing with her own toy – whether or not she's managed to grab hold of it yet. Though they are sitting near each other, they are not interacting.

TIME FOR A CHECK-UP

As with other aspects of development, the time that your baby will start to show particular signs of sociability cannot be given definitively. Probably even more than with other aspects of development, the timing of social milestones will vary from child to child. However, your baby will be increasingly responsive with every week that passes, and by eight weeks is likely to have started smiling. Over the coming weeks she will become excited when she sees you and will start to make verbal noises. The approximate timings given in this chapter should be used as a guide to development only. If you have any worries that your baby is not progressing as she should, you need to contact your child's pediatrician who can assess your child and discuss your concerns with you. In most cases, parents can be reassured about their worries and concerns but sometimes further assessments may be needed.

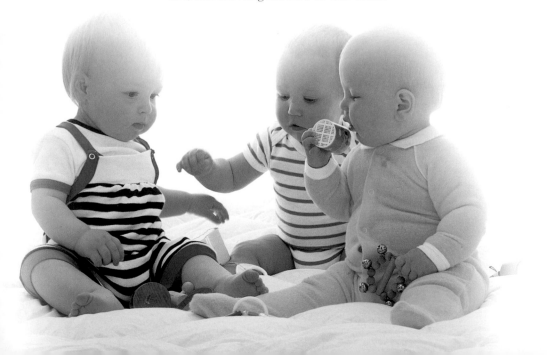

bonding

From the moment you meet your baby for the first time, a bond will begin to develop between you, which will strengthen with every day you spend together and will continue throughout your lives. In fact, this bonding process probably began even before your baby was born when you talked to him and stroked your abdomen. Although bonding is initiated by his parents, a child soon becomes a fully committed participant in the process.

Bonding is a vital part of your child's development. It is through establishing a secure and fulfilling relationship with his parents, that your child is able to go on and form satisfying friendships and romantic attachments, and be a welcome member of groups of all types. Bonding is also crucial for instilling in your child a basic trust in others that will help him form a model of how the social world functions and to understand how he fits in. There are serious consequences when a child does not have secure attachments in early life; he will fail to thrive both physically and emotionally.

How bonding occurs
Bonding is a natural process, which takes place in everything you do for your baby, from changing his diaper and soothing him when he cries, to reading him a story. By making your baby feel loved, safe, and secure you will strengthen his love for you and yours for him. In these first weeks and the months and years to come, there are countless things you will do for your baby that will make you close and strengthen the bond between you.

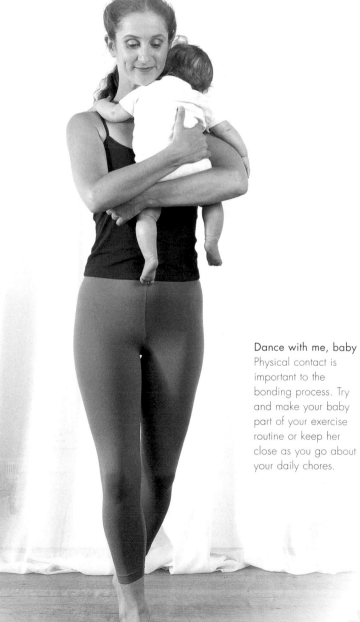

Dance with me, baby
Physical contact is important to the bonding process. Try and make your baby part of your exercise routine or keep her close as you go about your daily chores.

Bonding is based on communication and this is achieved in two main ways. The first is verbal, by talking and singing, and the other way is through physical contact.

Keep talking to your baby as you go about your daily activities. Even when he is small, your baby will love the sound of your voice so make sure you give him a running commentary on what you are doing and what is happening in the world around you.

Talk naturally to your baby. Even small babies pick up on the sounds and rhythm of words and normal conversation. Also, remember that communication is a two-way process; give your baby the opportunity to reply, even though for a year or more he won't say any words clearly. Respond to the sounds he makes with "Is that so?" or "I know." These positive responses will encourage him in his early attempts at language.

Babies love songs and music. Rocking your baby and dancing to music with him is something special that you can enjoy together. Front baby carriers or soft slings are great for keeping your baby close to you as you go about your daily routines.

Looking into your baby's face and smiling will make your baby feel close to you, so helping him to feel secure and content. Skin-to-skin contact and plenty of cuddles will also promote feelings of closeness and security.

Many women find that breastfeeding gives a special feeling of intimacy. It is this and the other benefits that make healthcare specialists recommend breast-feeding. However, if you decide to bottle-feed or find you are unable to breastfeed, do not feel that you are letting your baby down or that your bonding with him will be affected. You can come close to duplicating the experience by holding him next to your bare skin and making sure you maintain eye contact.

Your baby will not only communicate with you through the noises he makes and when he cries, he will also start to make gestures like holding his arms out to you when he wants to be picked up. Responding to these gestures will communicate to him that you understand and love him.

Your baby's contribution

Your baby is driven to obtain warmth, comfort, and security, from the earliest days of his life. He is, in fact, "pre-programed" to solicit responses from you. Immediately from birth, your baby will

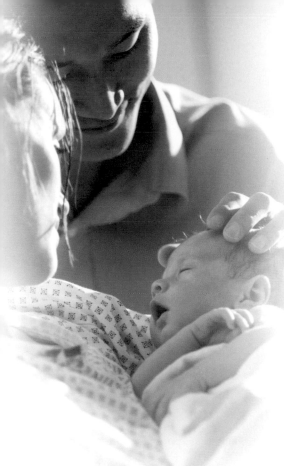

begin to communicate with those who care for and love him. He does this through crying, other noises, facial expressions, body movements, and touches.

As your baby grows, he'll learn how to predict your behavior, working out what will make you smile and encouraging you to pay attention to him. He smiles at you, stretches his arms out to your face so he'll be picked up, and snuggles into your neck when you cuddle him.

As he becomes more mobile, he'll still regard you as a secure base, seeking physical contact whenever he gets worried or afraid, or often just for the sheer joy of your response.

Other primary caregivers

You may feel that your partner has a head start in the bonding process; she spent nine months carrying your baby and then initially will spend almost every moment with him, particularly if she is breastfeeding. By talking to your baby and feeling his movements during the pregnancy and then being present when he is born, you will begin your close relationship with your child. Then, in everything you do with him and the time you spend together, the bond between you will strengthen.

If possible, take leave when your baby is born. This will ensure that you feel part of the early days when the bonding process begins, not only between you and your baby but also between the three of you as a family. If you are not able to take time off work, try to spend as much time as you can with your baby and your partner. Remember, bonding is not something that happens in the first few weeks of your baby's life but rather a closeness that will gradually grow over the coming months and years.

In the know... *Born to please*

Maternal and paternal feelings are inborn and normally do not require any learning or teaching. These feelings are triggered by certain features associated with a baby's appearance (which are also evident in adults and animals that we find hard to resist). Scientists have discovered that the following characteristics have a powerful appeal: A large head in relation to the body; a large, prominent, protruding forehead; large eyes set low down on the face; rounded, protruding cheeks; short, heavy limbs, with clumsy movements; a general plumpness and roundedness of the body – in short, the general appearance of a baby!

attachment

The bond that builds between you and your baby over the first months of her life means that she will soon come to rely on your being around. As a small baby, she may cope well with being passed from the arms of one eager relative to another, but with time she will come to feel safest with you and others with whom she has formed a close relationship. You will find that she is reluctant to be parted from you and may cry when you leave her and then smile when you come back. This separation anxiety classically tends to start around the age of seven months.

Attachment can be considered as a mechanism that manages the delicate balancing act between the survival of the young child and her need to explore and learn about her environment. How separations and reunions with caregivers are managed lead to a particular style of attachment developing between a child and each of her caregivers. The strength of your child's attachment to you can often be judged by the lengths that she will go in order to avoid separation, the exploration and withdrawal behaviors that occur when you are present, and the enthusiasm she shows when she is reunited with you.

The signs of attachment

Attachment develops to keep pace with mental skills.

* *As early as 3 months:* Your baby will become used to having you around and will probably start crying for your attention. Your response will comfort and settle her.

* *Around 4 months:* Your baby may start to cry when you leave the room. Over the coming months, she will become increasingly dependent on you for reassurance.

* *Around 6–8 months:* Your baby will start to show signs of stranger awareness. She also may want more cuddles and kisses.

* *Around 9–10 months:* Your baby will look up for you in a room to make sure you are still there.

TIME FOR A CHECK-UP

Shyness is common and, as we have already mentioned, many children never grow out of it completely. However it can usually be overcome sufficiently to enjoy social situations and live life to the fullest. If your child reaches the age of three years and her shyness is causing her problems – perhaps she always seems to be watching what is going on at child care rather than taking part, or maybe she is having problems making friends; in fact if you think her shyness is affecting her happiness in any way, it is important to talk to your child's pediatrician for advice. She may recommend ways to alleviate the problem and in a few cases may suggest counseling.

✳ *Around 18 months:* Your baby may be clingy and reluctant to be parted from you. Even a year or so later, she will continue to rely on you for reassurance and will still like to have you around, and until the age of three will, to a certain extent, rely on you for approval and reassurance.

✳ *Between 3 and 4 years:* She will be showing more signs of independence. Children of this age have to face being separated from their parents, perhaps at child care and then later at school. How your child reacts to this separation will depend partly on her personality but also on her previous experiences of caregivers and playing with other children.

✳ *By 4 years:* Children tend to be more independent and most are happy to be left for a time with familiar caregivers and then at child care and school.

Helping a baby or toddler to make the break

It is a good idea to let grandparents and trusted friends help to look after your baby from early on so that she gets used to having different people around her. This applies to babysitting, too; leaving a child's first babysitting experience until she is six months or more, when stranger awareness is developing, will make life more difficult for you and your baby.

Going to child care, too, will be easier if your child has had the experience of being cared for by others.

It is important to invite children to play; most children love having other children around to play and then going to their playmates' homes in return. At first, invite a parent along with a child, but once the child becomes familiar with you and

PARENTAL PARTICIPATION

It is important to give your baby the chance to spend time with other babies – she will really start to appreciate this from six months or so. Not only will she find it fun, but it will also help her to feel confident and safe in the company of others.

Join a playgroup

Many parks and centers offer opportunities for your child to play alongside or with others. Benefits include offering more activities than you can provide at home, such as sandboxes and water tables, but also gives you the opportunity to meet other parents.

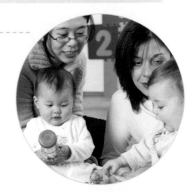

Take a class

Baby and toddler "gym," making music, baby massage, and movement classes are only some of the activities that are available for young children and their parents.

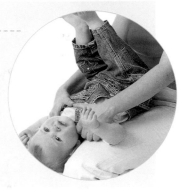

your home, she may be happy to remain unaccompanied. Strengthening your child's friendships will add to her confidence and help her to look forward to attending child care or school.

Your own separation anxiety

Your child is not the only one who will find separation difficult. Whenever it happens, whether you return to work and leave your child with a caregiver for the first time when she is a baby or whether the first prolonged separation comes later, this will be a difficult time for you, too. Talk to your caregiver – ask her to record what your baby does during the day, including what she plays with, what she eats, and any achievements made. Make sure you participate in your child's care every day as much as you can, whether this be giving her breakfast, bathing her, reading her a bedtime story, or giving a nighttime feeding.

Shyness

A three-month-old baby will be naturally outgoing and enjoy meeting new people. This will continue until the age of six months or so. Around this age babies are still friendly but may not be quite as out-going as they were previously. They also may need the reassurance of knowing a parent is there when they encounter someone who is not familiar to them. These are the first signs of the shyness that is to come. Over the next few months they will become increasingly aware of people they do not know. Your baby may now need to be encouraged to engage with a new person and may show her anxiety by holding on to you, and pressing her face against your shoulder.

This shyness is likely to continue for some time – an 18-month-old may still be clingy and look to her parent for reassurance. By the age of three, many children are still self-conscious and quiet around those who are unfamiliar to them or when they are in big groups.

As they get older, many children become more outgoing again; however, for some, signs of shyness persist and up to half of five- and six-years-olds still show some degree of shyness.

Aiding your child's progress

Building up your child's confidence and self-esteem will help her to overcome her shyness. There is nothing like a parent's love and appreciation of a child's efforts to boost confidence and feelings of self-worth, so give her plenty of attention and praise her frequently.

While there will be times when your child needs to be disciplined or shown her boundaries, try to be positive overall so that your child grows up in a positive, nurturing environment.

Never focus on shyness as a problem. This will only serve to make your child feel more self-conscious and worried about her social skills.

emerging emotions

A newborn cries when he is frustrated or uncomfortable and makes cooing noises when he is happy. With time, your baby learns to express his feelings in other ways; by his body movements as well as by his facial expressions, and ultimately through speech.

Behavioral scientists at the Gesell Institute discerned that from earliest infancy, children's emotions and behavior tend to alternate between periods of equilibrium and disequilibrium – primarily as a result of changes within their bodies, though environmental factors could help improve or exacerbate the situation. In other words, your child may fluctuate between periods when he is calm, happy, and contented, and those when he is moody, rebellious, and critical. If it helps you to be more sympathetic to your child's changes in temperament, bear in mind that the Gesell scientists believed that these fluctuations were necessary for greater emotional maturity.

The growth of emotional behavior

* *From around 1 month:* Your baby knows that you are his parents and will be reassured when you pick him up and talk to him. You will find that these simple actions will often settle him when he is crying. He will also turn to look at you when you speak close to him, and "talks" by jerking his body, moving his tongue and mouth, and nodding and bobbing his head.

* *Around 6 weeks:* Your baby will begin to show his contentment by smiling spontaneously. He also will start to anticipate and look forward to what is to come; for example, he may smile and make contented sounds as you get him ready for his bath.

* *Around 3 months:* He will start to giggle and squeal, kick his legs, and wave his arms when he is pleased. He will also

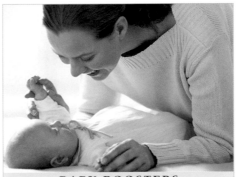

BABY BOOSTERS
SMILEY FACE

As with so many things, your baby will take your lead in learning to smile. Try to be a smiley person. Talk gently and positively when you are around your baby; make his environment a happy place to be. Try to remember that the sound of a harsh voice will upset him even though it is not directed at him.

make cooing noises and will start to shout out when he is happy or excited.

* *By 4–5 months:* Your baby will start to show his pleasure at seeing other people he recognizes by smiling. He will enjoy meeting new people and will smile at them, too. At around this age babies also begin to learn other facial expressions to let their parents know how they are feeling. Your baby will react differently to smiling and limit-setting.

* *Around 6 months:* Your baby may exhibit shyness with strangers by turning his face and body away or clinging to you. He has developed a comprehensive language to enable him to communicate through smiles, laughter, tears, cooing, and squealing as well as his body language.

* *Around 9 months:* This is the peak time for separation and stranger anxiety. Your baby will be upset when you leave and when strangers appear.

* *Around 1 year:* Your baby shows lots of affection by cuddling up to you. He will get angry if his toy is taken away and may become fearful of certain things – loud household appliances or animals, for example.

* *From 1 to 2 years:* Your toddler may display a temper, due to his inability to express himself in other ways. This should settle down and he'll become more easygoing and be able to express affection warmly by gestures and speech.

* *Around 2½ years:* This is a time when strong emotions take over as a result of frustration and insecurity brought on by your child's inability to do the things he wants to and his inability to contain and control his feelings.

* *Around 3 years:* Children exhibit different levels of being able to control their emotions. Some children have become calmer at this time while others still struggle with strong emotions. Some children are extremely confident; others fearful and insecure.

* *Around 4 years:* Your child may exhibit extremes of emotions – both positive and negative, loving certain things to excess, greatly disliking others.

* *At 5 years:* Generally positive in his outlook, calm, and serene, your child should have the maturity to take most troubles in stride.

Security objects

Most children need something – a blanket or soft toy – that reassures and comforts them. These "transitional objects" are vital to a child's emotional well-being and actually help them to become more independent.

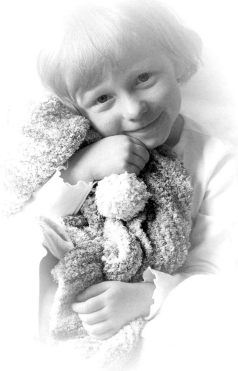

PARENTAL PARTICIPATION

Babies love to have fun and you will find many ways to make your baby giggle and laugh. As well as playing games like "Peekaboo" and "This Little Piggy," you can gently tickle him and blow raspberries against his skin.

Playing peekaboo

You can start to play this with your baby from the age of three to four months; however, once he has achieved object permanence (see page 78) at around nine months, he will enjoy this game much more. First try hiding behind your hands and then dropping them down. Next, you can hold a sheet in front of your baby and drop the sheet down so you can see his face. Give him big smiles and watch his joyful expression when he sees your face again.

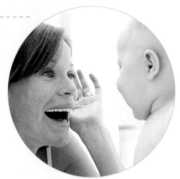

Having fun in the tub

Bath time is also an opportunity for fun. Gently splashing your baby and playing with the foam in the bath will make him giggle. He will love splashing in the water and getting everything wet – including you! You also can blow bubbles over the bath – at first he will enjoy simply watching them but later he will love trying to catch them. Waterproof books and bath toys also provide fun and learning opportunities while in the tub.

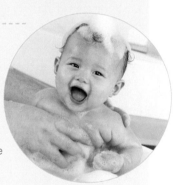

Singing nursery rhymes

Your baby will love to hear these simple songs again and again. He will really start to respond to them from six or seven months. However, it is never too early to start – even as a newborn, your baby will love the sound of your singsong voice and this special time you spend together. In addition to enjoying the music, he will learn language through the words you say. As he gets older, accompany the rhymes with some simple actions to entertain him – as in "The Itsy Bitsy Spider" – he will soon try to copy you.

moods

Children of any age can experience changes in mood. In young children, however, the reasons for these changes are likely to be easier to identify and to deal with. Young children also have difficulty in separating fantasy from reality, which can result in tearful episodes.

The first year

A baby's needs are relatively simple; she needs attention in the form of love and affection, food and drink, diaper changes, and entertainment. She also needs plenty of sleep. As long as these needs are met and she is healthy, your baby is likely to be content and happy. But, as soon as she is uncomfortable in any way, she will soon let you know by protesting with cries or screams. Her body language also will "tell" you whether she is content.

However, as all parents know, life is not always this simple. All babies will cry at some time for no apparent reason, but without knowing the reason, we can still usually calm them with simple measures such as rocking or singing. There is one particular exception to this and that is colic, the term used to describe the bouts of unexplained crying that some young babies experience, usually at the same time every day. Colic starts at about three weeks of age and continues until about three months of age. The reasons for colic are not known and, accordingly, we do not always know how to deal with the problem effectively.

Toddler times

For most toddlers, life is simple most of the time; things either go the way they want and they are happy, or they do not get their own way and they are tearful and frustrated. Whether toddlers are good-natured or grumpy also will be affected by their basic requirements – attention, sleep, food or drink, and entertainment.

The preschool child

As children get a little older and have an increasing awareness of those around them and of their own feelings, their moods may

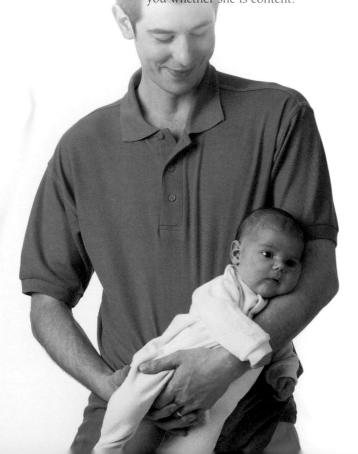

Stomach soother
Self-help measures for colic include laying your baby tummy down in your arms; the pressure against her abdomen may help to relieve the pain.

become a little more complex. Although the predominant mood in young children is still likely to be one of happiness and contentment, there may be times when your child will feel irritable. Often, such moods will be short-lasting and may again be related to tiredness, boredom, or hunger. However, in some cases, a mood of discontentment may have an underlying cause that needs to be addressed. It is up to parents to recognize these moods, and to provide help and support whenever it is needed.

A happy home

There are so many things you do to ensure your children remain happy and content, but the fundamental requirements are love and affection. Raising happy children also involves giving them a good deal of attention, while rewarding their attempts with praise and encouragement. As well as these basic needs, children also respond well to stability and a degree of routine.

When things go wrong

There will be times in most homes when things happen to disrupt the happy, stable atmosphere. Some may be unsettling only for a while, such as starting new child care or moving, during which extra attention, encouragement, and praise will be needed while your child settles back into a routine. But there may be more serious changes – such as relationship problems, bereavement, and financial troubles. Clearly no parent wishes to trouble or upset his or her children, but it can be hard for parents to consider the feelings of their children at all times when they are going through anguish and worry

---

In the know... *Colic*

Inconsolable crying or screaming, during which a baby may extend or pull up her legs and pass gas, is known as colic. About one-fifth of babies develop it, usually between the second and fourth weeks of life. Although most colic disappears by around three months, you should consult your child's pediatrician to rule out any medical reason such as hernia or gastroesophageal reflux disorder (GERD).

---

themselves. It is important during these troubled times that parents seek as much help and support as they need.

A happy child is likely to look well, eat well, and play well. Children are like this most of the time. However, even quite young children can become upset and worried about things. Obvious signs of this may be a change from your child's usual sleeping pattern or poor eating. You also may notice your child is not as outgoing as she usually is or is reluctant to go to child care. She may seem sad sometimes or may be more irritable and grumpy than usual. No one knows your child better than you do. If you see any signs that there is a problem and you are not able to get to the root of it yourself, see your child's pediatrician for advice.

Vivid imaginations

Young children are blessed with vivid imaginations; it is in fantasy play that they often explore and come to terms with a wide range of emotions. Sometimes, however, this make-believe world becomes a little too real, and a child becomes upset or frightened by some element of imaginary play – a monster out of control or an accident to an imaginary friend. Fantasy play is important to your child's development, so don't belittle or make fun of these incidents. Instead, try to join in and solve the problem – help chase the monster away – but then let your child continue to manage her fantasy play as she'd like.

Grumpy phases

You can sometimes feel that nothing you say or do is right when your four year old contradicts you at every turn. This does not mean that you are doing anything wrong, just that your child is going through an irritable phase. Often this will coincide with times of change when she is feeling unsettled. Tiredness may also be a factor. Sometimes, children go through such phases for no apparent reason, and

Irritability
While toddlers and young children tend to spend most of their time being happy and contented, like us they can be irritable and bad-tempered. If your child is feeling grumpy, you will soon know about it.

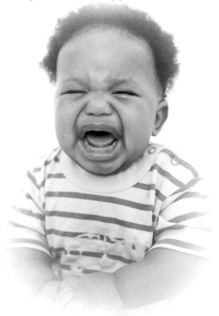

In the know... *Imaginary friends*

Many young children have imaginary friends. Some have a single, long-term companion or pet, others many, different, shorter-lasting ones. They do not mean a child is shy or in some way maladjusted; in fact, scientists believe that they can help a child become better adjusted and more able to cope with stress.

Because imaginary companions can help a child to experiment with different emotions – particularly "forbidden feelings" – and experiences, it's a good idea for parents to "play along with" and even encourage these imaginary friends, perhaps by supplying a few props for the "friend" to play with.

---

the mood will lift as suddenly as it began. Like adults, children can seem to get out of bed on the wrong side for no apparent reason. If your child is in a grumpy mood, keep smiling and be positive, encouraging her to get on with her day.

Irritability in the short-term may be related to being hungry. It also may be that your child has had a poor night's sleep and needs to rest for an hour or two. However, irritability also may indicate that she has something on her mind. Talking to her generally about what she has been doing at child care and maybe asking her specific questions about friends at preschool may uncover something to explain her mood.

Remember, if your child continues to be irritable, bad-tempered, or unhappy, see your child's pediatrician for advice.

anger and aggression

Like all of us, toddlers can become angry and frustrated at times. They can show this in many ways. Angry feelings can manifest themselves as tantrums, angry outbursts that typically begin at about two years of age. An angry child may bang his fists on the table or throw objects across the room. Anger and frustration can also be expressed as aggressive behavior like hitting or kicking.

Frustration

Toddlers can easily become frustrated and it is no accident that the most extreme forms of this frustration, tantrums, may begin as early as 15 months.

Toddlers have to live with certain physical limitations – they may not be able to move around as fast as they would like or be dexterous enough to play as they would wish. Their speech is limited, too, so they may not be able to make their parents understand what they want. Children of this age also are showing the early signs of independence and wanting to take some control of what is happening to them.

Tantrums

These outbursts are very common and are experienced by most toddlers. They are most common around the age of two, but can occur in children as young as 15–18 months and as old as four years or more.

The most important thing for a parent to remember is to keep calm, no matter how hard this may be. Remember, this behavior is normal and reflects your child's frustration, at not being physically able to do something, not being able to make himself understood, feeling he doesn't have

your attention, or sometimes at just not being able to get his own way.

If a tantrum occurs, you can try to offer your child some comfort by hugging him but if you find your child struggles or is hard to contain, try ignoring the behavior. Stay calm and continue with what you are

Try a cuddle
In the early stages of a tantrum, a young child may be soothed by some hugs and kisses.

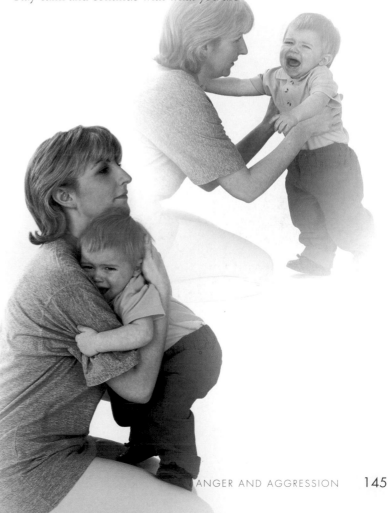

doing. In addition to ignoring inappropriate behavior, immediately attend to and praise appropriate behavior.

Make sure your child is positioned safely so that he will not hurt himself if he punches and kicks. If you catch the tantrum early enough you may be able to distract your child.

Toddlers often pick locations where they have an audience for their shows – the more people that are around, the worse the behavior is likely to be. If your child has a tantrum when you are on an outing, you may not feel able to ignore the behavior for long. If the tantrum starts to gather momentum and your child cannot be distracted, carry him away from his audience to somewhere you can be more or less on your own. In as few words as possible, explain to him what you are doing calmly and quietly. Place him down safely and wait patiently for him to calm. This may take five minutes or even longer. Don't worry – and keep your resolve. You do not want your child to believe that he can get what he wants through throwing a tantrum.

Try to preempt your child's frustration.

❋ *Look out for factors that may be fueling his anger:* Is he tired, hungry, or bored, for instance? Is he getting enough opportunities to blow off steam and stop tensions building up? (Take him outside every day at least once to run around.)

❋ *Make efforts to understand him:* Often you will not be able to understand what he wants, but do your best.

❋ *Praise him when he behaves well:* Use words as rewards; don't buy him treats as this will set a precedent. Toddlers respond well to positive reinforcement.

❋ *Remember your child is an individual:* Different approaches suit different children. You will need to find what works for your child.

Aggressive behavior

Anger and frustration, sometimes fueled by jealousy (which is common in toddlers), may sometimes be expressed in the form of aggression, perhaps as hitting, hair pulling, or even biting. You need to be firm on this; let your toddler know that it

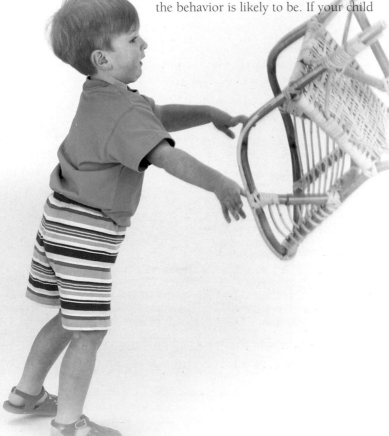

Distruptive behavior
Your child may be using unsocial acts in order to call attention to his needs.

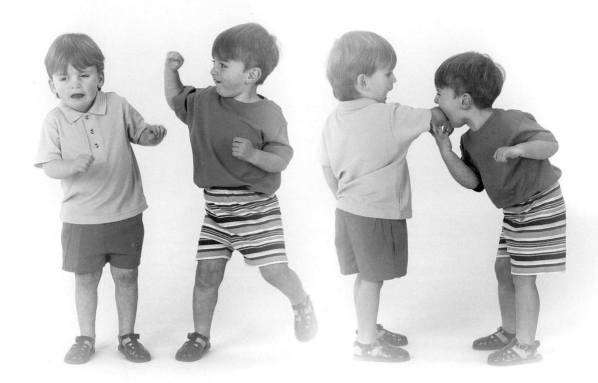

is normal to be angry but not to hurt others in any way. A few tips are:

＊ Don't ignore the fact that he is angry: Talk to him about his feelings.

＊ Offer to give him a hug when he is ready: It will make you feel better, too.

＊ Don't be hurt if your toddler lashes out at you occasionally: This is not personal and does not reflect on your relationship or your parenting skills. Most parents will experience this at sometime or another.

＊ Be firm: Say "No" when your child oversteps the mark.

How to keep your cool

As any parent will find out, this is not easy when you are faced with difficult behavior. Your child will occasionally be a source of frustration for many years to come. These are just a few tips to help you stay calm:

＊ Take a break: In the short term, step away from your child and take some deep breaths. Explain that you are angry and that this is helping you. In this way you are also showing your child that everyone gets angry and that anger does not have to be expressed through aggression.

Also, if possible, plan an evening or a few hours out without your child.

＊ Go easy on yourself: Do not constantly berate yourself when you are feeling angry and frustrated. It is normal to feel angry – the important thing is knowing how to manage it by finding ways to calm down; perhaps making yourself a cup of tea or putting on some music.

＊ Talk about it: Sharing your frustrations and worries with a sympathetic friend or relative will help.

＊ Be reasonable: Limit the number of times you have to say "No." Use other forms of discipline like redirection, ignoring behavior, or humor.

＊ Stay positive: Focus on the good in your child; celebrate this and deal with negative behavior consistently and fairly.

Bullying

Toddlers may act on aggressive feelings by biting or abusing a playmate. You need to take steps to nip such behavior in the bud.

play

Play makes a vital contribution to every child's development; it is through play that children learn new skills and then rehearse them for adult life. As well as helping to improve motor (movement) skills, coordination, and mental skills like reasoning, play helps children to develop and practice their social skills. Play also allows children to express their individuality as well as to understand and express emotions through imaginary play.

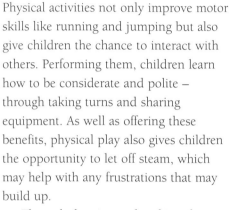

Letting off steam
Toddlers of around two years and more are particularly prone to becoming frustrated and they, like older children, need the opportunity to run around and play in the fresh air.

The importance of play to sociability

Any time spent playing is valuable time. Various types of play help different aspects of development and learning, such as building physical and mental skills, but all types of play can give a child the opportunity to learn about relationships and getting along with other children.

Physical activities not only improve motor skills like running and jumping but also give children the chance to interact with others. Performing them, children learn how to be considerate and polite – through taking turns and sharing equipment. As well as offering these benefits, physical play also gives children the opportunity to let off steam, which may help with any frustrations that may build up.

Through drawing and making things, children are able to express their individuality. Such creative activities also help to build a child's confidence and self-esteem. Sharing materials such as crayons and glue is often a part of this play.

In experimenting with toys such as stacking blocks and shape sorters, children come to understand more about the world around them and how things work. As they get older, children enjoy making their discoveries together.

However, it is through "pretend" play that children probably learn more about social interaction and behavior than through any other type of play. Pretend play emerges around 18 months to two years of age and becomes increasingly

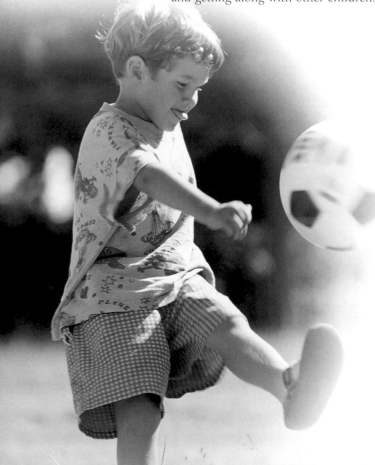

more complex over time. Role play with other children and with dolls and stuffed animals gives children the opportunity to learn about relationships and social interaction. They find out about caring for others and taking the feelings of others into consideration in their everyday lives.

How children play

The way children play changes as they get older. They begin with solitary play, moving to playing alongside others (parallel play), and finally to full engagement with others or associative and cooperative play.

Although babies are not capable of playing with other children, they love to be in their company and to watch them playing. Toward the end of their first year, babies may take an interest in the things with which another child is playing, and may grab interesting objects or toys but they are not really playing with another child of a similar age.

Toddlers are happy to play alongside others but are still looking to an adult for "approval" of their behavior and generally will not interact with another child if their parents aren't present. This playing alongside is known as parallel play and it continues until the age of two to three years, when children start to play more interactively.

Two- to five-year-olds normally use all forms of play at some time during the day. Your three-year-old, for example, may occupy herself with solitary play with a doll, may later play alongside a friend with her own toys, which can lead to associative play – where she swaps toys or materials with this other child, but indulges in her

PARENTAL PARTICIPATION

As a parent, one of your key roles regarding play is to provide a stimulating environment for it to take place. Children need very little equipment for imaginary play but you may like to provide the following.

Store-bought sets

A tea set, a doctor's set, or a tool kit will provide your toddler and young child with lots of imaginative play opportunities.

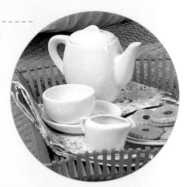

Useful household items

Many common items such as a hairbrush and comb, kitchen utensils such as a whisk and plastic bowl, and cleaning materials such as brooms provide scope for domestic role playing. Remember though to only offer safe items.

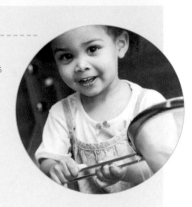

Pretend store

In addition to store-bought play cash registers, shopping can be brought to life with perhaps a few shoe boxes and pairs of shoes, or some cans of food and a basket.

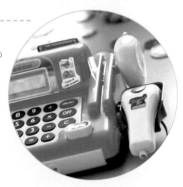

own play – and finally engage in fully cooperative play or games. Although babies and young toddlers are not capable of associative or cooperative play with other children, such play is part and parcel of the daily activities of parent and child – dressing, feeding, and diaper changing. While this "play" is not exactly the same as with another child, it indicates that very young children are perfectly used to collaborative kinds of play, although actually doing it with a child of the same age is not possible until a certain developmental stage has been achieved.

Once young children play together, they are likely to disagree – frequently if they are strong-willed. One key cause for this is an unwillingness to share. You may spend many a frustrating afternoon refereeing such disagreements. Bear in mind, until the age of about three, children do not begin to understand the concepts of sharing or taking turns. Even

Playing games
Children may be able to learn to play simple card games from the age of four and in some cases earlier. These are great for learning numbers and other key information as well as taking turns and listening to others.

In the know... Gender games
Through role playing, children explore the nature of what it means to be male or female. Children are very susceptible to the influence of television and other media, and the attitudes of friends and relations. Even if both parents work and share family responsibilities equally, a child still may persist in acting out conventional gender roles – a girl will want to wear make-up and play house, while a boy may run around with a light saber. On the other hand, some children go against gender types. A girl may become very aggresive or a boy put on his sister's clothes. It is through experimenting with the attitudes and behaviors of both sexes that children gain a firm idea of their own.

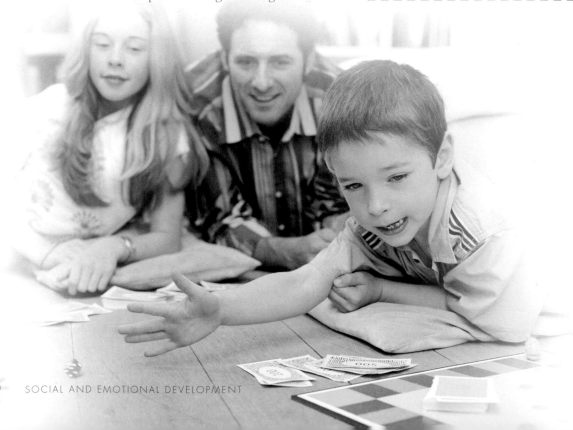

when children eventually learn to share well, it does not mean they will always do it (see page 154 for advice on sharing).

From the age of four or so, children start to understand each other's point of view so they may become able to reach compromises and to consider each other's wishes as they play.

Helping your child to play

It is important to let children take the lead as often as possible during all types of play, particularly pretend and creative play. Interfering and taking over will only curb a child's natural imagination and creativity. Part of the fun of fantasy play for children is that they are able to control their imaginary dramas. They feel in control of things. Younger children, however, may welcome help, and there may be times when you feel fantasy play could help your child deal with a worry that she has. In this case, you could suggest a scenario, for example, if you're leaving her with a babysitter, you might suggest she plays babysitter with her doll. But even if you are asked to join in, you should keep a low profile. Your main job is to do what your child suggests and not to take over the play. You should give only as much help as is needed.

By playing with your child you can teach her important skills, not only how to do things practically, but also about taking turns and sharing. However, she will also learn a great deal from amusing herself sometimes, knowing that you are around if she needs you. Playing on her own for short periods will make your toddler feel in control of what is happening around her and will boost her self-confidence.

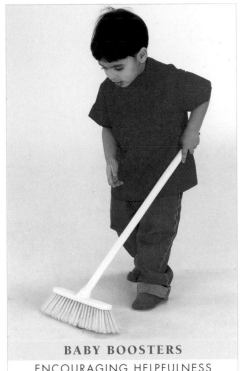

BABY BOOSTERS
ENCOURAGING HELPFULNESS

Even young children should be encouraged to participate in "clean up time'" after a play session. This is all part of learning to be helpful as well as to respect and take care of things. You can make this a fun part of a play session by giving your child his own safe cleaning materials or by asking your child to collect all the same type or color of toys together and put them in the box for you, or by counting or singing as you work.

party, party

Parties are a great way for your child to socialize with friends. However, it won't be until the age of three that he'll fully understand what a party is, though at age two, he'll be able to appreciate the specialness of the occasion.

Prepare your toddler for the party by talking about it to him a few days in advance, and discussing who's coming. Your older child may be able to help with the invitations and some simple food preparation. Many older children will have clear ideas about who they want to invite and what kind of party they want – one with a pirate theme or a jewelry-making afternoon, for example.

Keep the menu simple. Serving healthy snacks in addition to the traditional cake and ice cream is a good idea. And offer milk or water as a beverage, instead of juice or soda.

Two-year-olds

Toddlers of this age will only enjoy a party of a short duration – about an hour is usually sufficient and with only a few friends. It's a good idea to invite the guests' parents to stay, as children of this age are not that sociable and generally will want to play in the presence of their parents. Have fun, age-appropriate activities planned for the children and their parents.

Three-year-olds

Older toddlers can tolerate a party of about one-and-a-half hours. Keep the guest list to about six children. Make sure you've allowed for solitary play with a selection of your child's toys as well as some simple group activities, like grab-bag party favor selection. The children will be too young to play

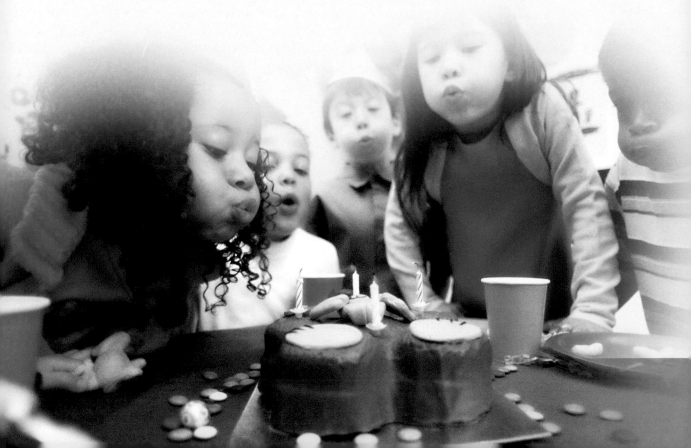

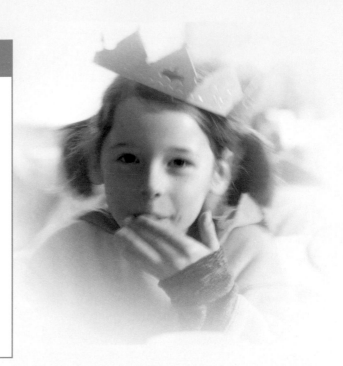

- Reserve one area in which to serve food and for quiet play and another area for more boisterous activities.
- Cover the floor under the party table with plastic and only half fill cups to prevent spills.
- Stock up on wet wipes and paper towels for mopping up spills and cleaning sticky hands and faces.
- Keep a supply of spare pants on hand in case of accidents. Remind the children to use the potty as with the excitement, they might forget.
- Put away any toys your child doesn't want to share.

party games but may enjoy simple action songs, such as "Ring-Around-the-Rosy" or being allowed to use backyard play equipment.

Four-year-olds

At this age your child will really love a party. Still keep the numbers small – six to eight guests are sufficient and the time short – one-and-a-half to two hours at most. Make sure you have some toys, dressing up items, or favors available for play and keep organized games to a minimum. Most children will enjoy games with music like "Musical Chairs." Try to arrange it so every child wins a prize.

Five-year-olds

Parties for children of this age need planning as they will be most successful when there is structured activity. The excess energy that five-

year-olds display also must be catered to, generally by some periods of more active play. Because children of this age still find it hard to take turns, you should still keep numbers small. Plan on a party of two hours. In addition to organized games and/or entertainment, make sure children have things to play with from the beginning while other guests arrive and after the cake, when they are waiting to be picked up.

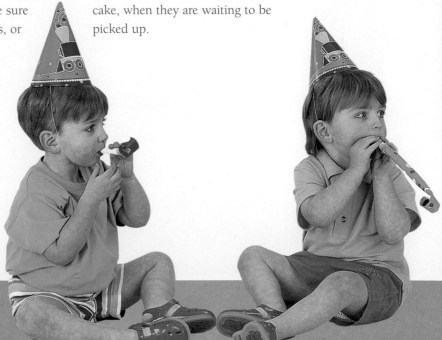

sharing

Most children start learning to share some time after the age of three. By four, they should have a good, but not infallible, understanding of the concept and fallings-out with playmates over particular toys should become less frequent. You can help the learning process along by asking your child's playmates to come and play in your home so that your child is asked to share her toys sometimes.

How it happens

Before children come to understand sharing, they learn about owning things. Your toddler will go through a phase when she will describe all sorts of things as being hers – not only her own possessions but everyone else's. By the age of two, she will probably have come to realize that although some things are hers, others belong to other people. (You can help her understand this by pointing at things, saying "Daddy's shoes," "Mommy's nose.") Appreciating this is the first step in coming to grips with sharing.

How to help your child

Learning to share and take turns is a natural progression in child development. However, there are a number of measures you can take to help things along and hopefully make for a more harmonious atmosphere.

While your toddler needs to learn about sharing her toys, always ask her whether her friend can play with one; never presume she will agree and never hand the toy over if she refuses. Making her share her possessions against her wishes will only upset her and make her

Give it here
Young toddlers don't feel any guilt about grabbing what they want. Their lack of awareness of the feelings of others means they can be very physical at times.

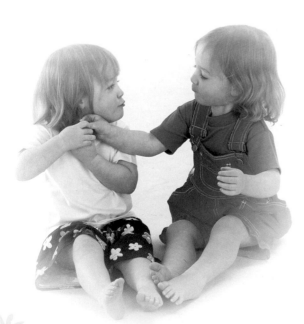
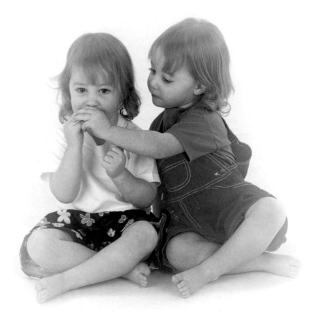

more resistant to sharing next time. When your toddler does let a sibling or friend play with one of her toys, praise her enthusiastically. Never get angry with your toddler for refusing to share. Remember, this is normal for a child of her age.

Be fair. Don't always make your child give her toys up for a visiting child; the same applies to siblings – don't always expect an older child to be the "sensible one" and give up her toys for her younger sibling. Don't rush in to pass a ruling on which child should have a particular toy – give children an opportunity to come to an agreement on their own first.

Try to avoid confrontation. If your child has a particular toy that she and her friend always fight over, perhaps a doll or a dressing-up outfit, ask the visitor to bring her own along. This will help to create a happy environment where other toys are more likely to be shared.

Your toddler also must learn to share toys provided for everyone to share, for example, equipment in a playground or

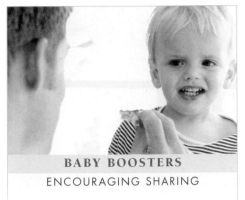

BABY BOOSTERS
ENCOURAGING SHARING

If you want your child to learn to share, you need to set her a good example. Make sure you share your own possessions with your toddler sometimes and that she sees you doing so with others.

musical instruments in a singing class. After she has had a reasonable turn on the swings or maracas, show her that another child is waiting and interest her in doing something else. Set a timer for five minutes. Each child gets a turn with the toy and has to trade when the timer rings.

Sharing a parent

As well as having to learn to share toys and other possessions, children have to learn to share their parents with others, whether this be other adults or a younger sibling, or even chores that need doing. Toddlers need to understand that they cannot always be the focus of attention for their parents who may want to spend time with others or who have their own activities to fit into the day.

A child, particularly a first child, may find it hard to let her parent visit with others or to do her everyday tasks rather than playing. If you experience this, there

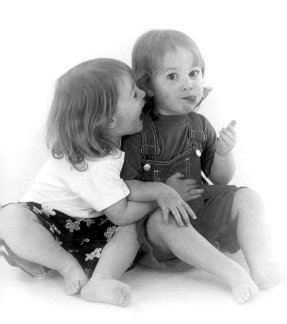

are a few simple things you can try to help your child with this.

* ***When she is a baby:*** Position her chair so that she can see what you are doing.
* ***As she gets older, involve her in your activities:*** If you are dusting, give her a cloth; if you are doing the laundry, let her help you put the clothes in the machine; if you are writing a shopping list, ask her to make her own list by scribbling, or if she is older, by drawing the things you need.
* ***Give her quality time:*** When you do an activity with her, make her the focus of your attention.
* ***Avoid repeatedly stalling:*** Explain what you are going to do and when you will be able to play with her.

Mixed blessings
A toddler may have conflicting feelings about a new sibling. Try to get your older child involved with your new one but also spend time alone with your toddler.

* ***Keep your promises:*** If you say you will play with her when you have finished the laundry, try your best to do it.
* ***Don't feel guilty:*** Provided she has your company, it is good for your toddler to learn how to amuse herself. No parent can be a playmate every minute of the day.

A new sibling

It is often very hard for a young child to share her parents with a new brother or sister. For some time, she will have been the main focus of their attention and now a baby, who seems to do little but cry and sleep, is taking her parents' attention away from her. If you are going to have a second child, it is important to make preparations so that your child is as ready as she can be. Key to this is making her feel involved. Talk to her about the baby. Take her with you when you go shopping, and let her choose a small present to give the new baby. When the baby is born, make sure your young child sees you and the new baby before anyone else so she is part of this special time. Giving her a present from the baby will also help.

Once you are home, ask your child to help you look after the baby. Give her simple tasks like asking her to bring you a diaper, then praise her for being such a good helper. Remember that she still needs some one-to-one time with you. Try to make opportunities for this every day – read her a bedtime story or do one of her favorite activities with her while someone else looks after the baby. As your first child gets older, it is important to remember that she will still appreciate time that is just for her, particularly as she will be interested in activities that will be unsuitable for your younger child.

empathy

To a toddler, the world and those around him exist for his comfort and entertainment. This egocentrism is universal in toddlers and is shown when they refuse to share, refuse to take turns, or refuse to wait for a parent to do something for them. Gradually, the realization will come that the world does not revolve around this one, small person and that the feelings of others need to be taken into consideration.

The waiting game

Your toddler will expect everything to be done now, this minute, no matter what you are doing, be it driving, talking on the telephone, preparing the family meal, or going to the bathroom. Immediate action is not always possible and gradually you will teach your child that he is not the only one with needs and wishes.

When your toddler makes a request, encourage him to be polite as soon as he is able – this is one important part of learning to be considerate toward others.

At first, he will only be able to point at what he wants, or say the odd word, but as soon as he is talking, encourage him to ask pleasantly.

Although you may not be able to follow his wishes right away, do respond to your child promptly. Ignoring him, no matter how valid the reason seems, will only serve to frustrate and upset him. If you can help him immediately sometimes, do so – there will be plenty of times when this will not be possible and when, therefore, you will be teaching him to wait.

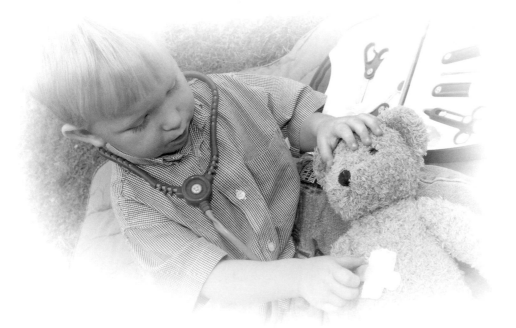

How does it feel?
Role playing caring jobs is a way that children learn how others are feeling.

Avoid repeatedly stalling by saying "in a minute." It is all too easy to do this, but these delays will be frustrating for him. Furthermore, small children have no idea what time or the future means – you may as well say you'll help him in one hour or one day. Instead, explain what you are doing and that when this task is completed, you will help him. If possible, suggest something he can do while you finish what you are doing or involve him in your own task. Stick to your promises so that your child knows he can rely on what you say.

Sometimes your toddler's request may be unnecessary, for example, asking you to pass something to him when it is well within his reach. Encourage your child to help himself and praise him when he does.

Caring play

Through playing with dolls and stuffed animals, young children practice the caring role. This type of "pretend" play tends to start between the ages of two and three years. All children need for this is a doll or stuffed animal, a tea set, a blanket to put the "baby" to sleep, doll's clothes and perhaps a doctor's set. Your child also will be happy to learn through looking after you, perhaps making you a pretend cup of coffee, brushing your hair, or simply patting your head if it hurts.

Being kind

You may feel upset that your toddler seems to be unkind to other children sometimes. This is normal; as we have said, young

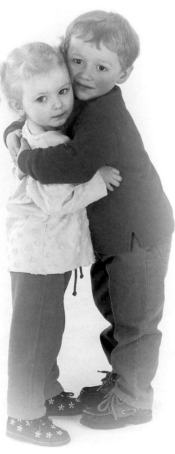

Making up
Toddlers sometimes have to be persuaded to say "Sorry" for aggressive actions but in no time they can be friends again.

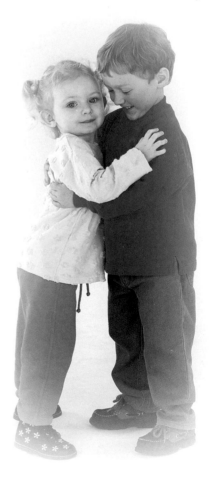

children cannot appreciate the feelings of others, and are fully occupied with thoughts of themselves. As they develop empathy, the ability to share and take turns becomes easier.

Remember, kindness is something your child will learn about from your example. Being polite, kind, and considerate toward others yourself will create the right environment for your child to develop these qualities. You can make him a part of a kind act, for example, by suggesting you make a card together for someone who is sick, or do an errand together for a housebound neighbor.

Don't expect too much from your young toddler and feel let down if he pushes another child or refuses to share.

TIME FOR A CHECK-UP

All toddlers can be unkind and even aggressive toward others at times. This is a normal part of development that will pass. However, if your child's behavior seems to be unreasonable to you or is affecting her relationships with other children, seek advice from your child's pediatrician. Occasionally, such extremes of behavior reflect an underlying problem that needs to be addressed.

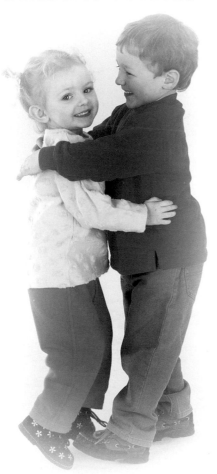

Remember, this is all part of the learning process and he is making progress all the time. The reaction from the other child will inform this process and help your child come to realize that he is being unreasonable. However, there should be a consequence for aggressive or hurtful behavior. Around age two, a "time-out" (see page 191) for selective negative behaviors can be initiated.

Never force your toddler to be kind by handing his toys over to another child without asking him or letting a child go before him at the playground when it is his turn. The learning process will work best if he is encouraged to be kind and considerate on his own.

Sharing feelings

While you do not want to burden a child with your troubles, there is no harm in telling him in a matter-of-fact way how you are feeling sometimes. Telling him you are tired or hungry will help to develop his awareness of the feelings of others.

Getting older and wiser

Empathy develops over time, although it may be apparent early on. A young baby, for example, not only cries because he isn't "happy," he may cry if he sees his mother do so.

* **Around 2 years:** Children start to interact with each other more during play. Although, at this stage, they remain unaware of their playmates' points of view, they may respond to another person's distress by becoming distressed themselves. Over the next two years they will start to consider the feelings of others.

* **Around 3 years:** Your child will show that he understands another person's situation rather than relating it to his own experience, for example, by seeking out your help if he sees a younger sibling cry.

* **Around 4 years:** He will be able to consider conflicting emotions before responding – pleasure, if his younger sibling is reprimanded for taking his toys but sympathy when he or she bursts into tears. He also will be more able to wait for things to happen as he gains more of an understanding of what is going on around him and that not everything that happens relates to him.

* **Around 5 years:** Children are able to appreciate the needs and wishes of others, although this does not necessarily mean they will put the needs of others before their own. Children of this age become concerned about their siblings and friends. They will take care of their younger brothers and sisters, perhaps holding their hands protectively when they enter a room of children or an unfamiliar place.

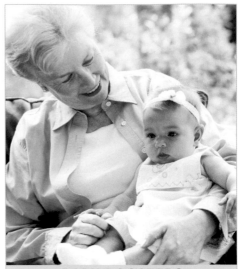

BABY BOOSTERS
BUILDING RELATIONSHIPS

The grandparent-grandchild relationship can be vital to a child's development. If you live nearby, you should take advantage of opportunities to be part of your grandchild's activities and interests. And you may develop games or go on outings that are special for just the two of you. If this isn't possible, you can maintain the relationship by keeping in frequent contact – through the telephone, mail, and even e-mail. Exchanging photos can keep you both abreast of what is happening in your lives.

Developing an understanding of the perspective of others may come earlier if children have siblings or if they spend time with groups of children, perhaps at child care.

temperament

The development of personality depends on nature and nurture – the genes we inherit from our parents and the environment in which we live, in particular how we are brought up. These two vital factors interact to form the unique individuals we are.

During the early years of life, changes in temperament and behavior occur that are not unique to individuals but form a recognized part of normal development. As a child gets older and her personality develops, certain aspects of her temperament will become more constant and more obvious to those around her.

The early years

All children tend to show certain aspects of sociability at particular ages, for example, smiling usually begins at around the age of six weeks and addressing parents as "Mommy" and "Daddy" by the age of two. They also tend to show certain types of behavior at particular ages. For example, up to the age of about seven or eight months, babies tend to be outgoing and gregarious; then they become more reserved for a while, holding back when they meet new people. From around the age of two, many children become easily frustrated and impatient with parents and others who cannot understand what they are trying to say, or say "No" to their demands. Two-year-olds also can become frustrated by their own physical limitations. These frustrations can lead to aggressive behavior and, in many cases, tantrums. By the age of four years,

children are likely to be more patient; they are more articulate and have started to develop insight into the feelings of others, and to learn about the art of reasoning. However, they are still likely to be quarrelsome at times and to fight with their friends as they all try to exert their independence.

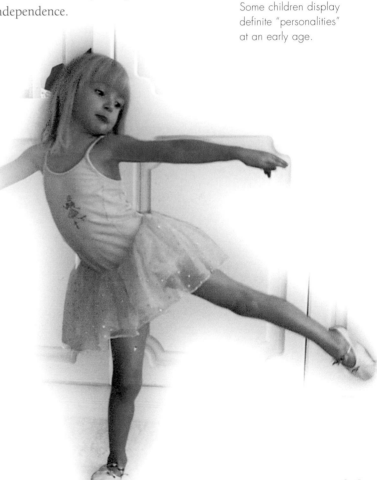

Future dancer
Some children display definite "personalities" at an early age.

By the age of five, individual personality traits start to become apparent. You will notice that some five-year-olds are more patient than others, some are more extroverted than others, and some are more caring than others. These are by no means absolute indicators in terms of future personality, but they do give some insight into the type of person a child is likely to be.

What determines personality

Certain aspects of our personality are programmed when we are born as a result of our genes. However, the way we are brought up and treated by others will influence these features and how they manifest themselves as we get older. As parents, you want to provide the best environment you possibly can to nurture your children and help them to reach their full potential. However, the effects you have on their personalities will have limits.

– – – – – – – – – – – – – – – – – –

In the know...Personality

It used to be thought that once developed, personality remained the same throughout life. Scientists no longer believe this is true. In fact, as people get older they begin to change at an accelerated rate. Our inherited traits begin to change and accommodate to different surroundings and experiences. You may be surprised when your boisterous and booming toddler becomes a quiet and hardworking schoolchild.

– – – – – – – – – – – – – – – – – –

In other words, a child's personality and how she will respond to the world around her is, to a certain extent, preordained, and parental influence can only go so far. As parents, understanding this should relieve you of some of the pressure at times when your children do not behave as you would wish them to.

It is because of the differences in genes and temperament traits between individuals that two children brought up in the same way will show differences in personality; one may be reserved and quiet, the other talkative and outgoing; one may sleep well, the other get up during the night and wake early.

Making comparisons

Remember that your child has inherited a mix of genes, half from you and half from your partner. This mix makes her an individual who may be like one or both of you in some respects but may also be very different from both of you. This applies not only to how she looks but also to her temperament. Do not expect your child to be outgoing because you are, or ambitious because you have a high-level job. Avoid making comparisons and feeling disappointed that your child is different from you; celebrate the differences – they are what makes her the special individual that she is.

Giving labels

While it may be helpful to recognize particular features of your child's temperament to help parent your child appropriately and anticipate her needs, it is not thought to be helpful to label a child as having a particular personality trait. A

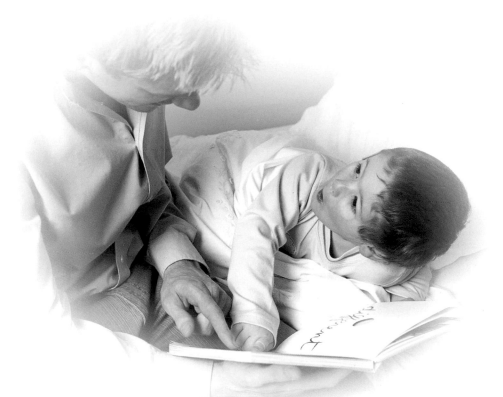

Avoiding battles
Some children need more wind-down time than others. Find ways of fitting in with your child's personality so that both of you will enjoy everyday routines.

child's personality is still developing, and hearing herself described in a certain way may upset her and also may make her live up to the description. In addition, having made an assessment of your child's personality, you also may subscribe to this opinion and be too rigid in how you manage your child's behavior.

Understanding your child

Learning to understand and accept the temperament of your child is an important stage in nurturing her personality and helping her to fit in with the world around her. For example, if your child is reluctant to go to parties or to a friend's house to play, you can develop strategies to prepare her and give her the confidence to cope with the situation. Also, instead of being disappointed or blaming yourself when things seem to go wrong, you can move on in a positive way to deal with any problems that may arise.

Developing a strategy

Strive to understand your child's temperament and focus on her strengths. A "strong-willed" child has perseverance. Give her challenging toys to manipulate and analyze. Dealing with her temperament in a positive way allows her to thrive. Take a step back and look at who your child is. Sometimes, the child who is most like you can be the most challenging to deal with.

all about me

Making a scrapbook about your child is a great project for both of you. Not only are you creating a precious family keepsake, but you'll be helping your child to see himself as an individual. Scrapbooking is a wonderful, easy parent/child activity that should have you smiling and laughing the whole time. It's also something that you can return to again and again in case your child gets easily bored (see box for some simple ideas).

The book should center on your child's friends and family, holidays and activities, favorite things and interests. By helping to make the book, your child will be using a number of skills. He should be encouraged to talk about the things he wants to include – and possibly write some labels – and also to provide drawings.

Explain to your child that you are going to create a book about him and that you are going to use photographs, pictures, postcards, and his

SIMPLE SCRAPBOOKING PROJECTS

- Create a family tree with your child. Show him how the tree starts with his grandparents (or great-grandparents) and then branches out to include his parents, aunts and uncles, and cousins.
- Make a day in the life of your child. Take photos from when he wakes up to when he goes to bed. If he can handle it, give him a disposable camera to take some pictures of things he finds memorable.
- Take handprints of your child at regular stages to show him how he grows. Use waterproof ink and a roller.
- Make a birthday book where each page or two details a particular year – the party photos, vacations, accomplishments.

drawings. Ask him to think about how he would describe himself and the things that are important to him. If he's not sure what you mean, you can prompt him by saying "Would you like to put in some photos of last summer's vacation at the beach?" or "Should we use this picture of you and

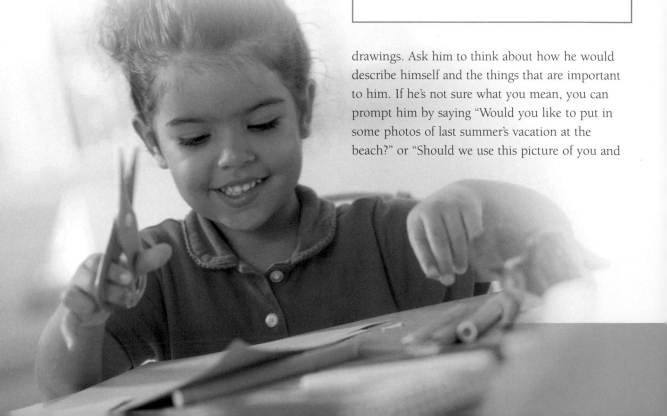

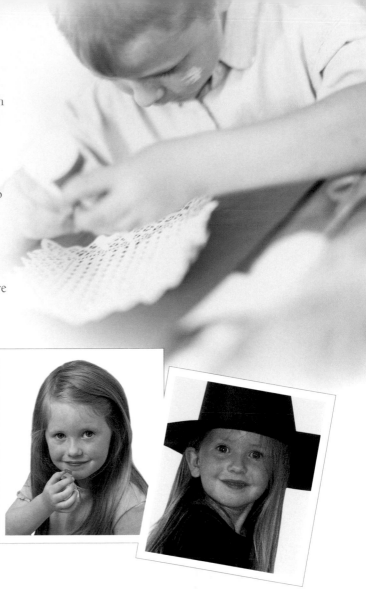

Grandma?" Ask him to name his favorite foods, colors, storybook characters, and games. Sit down and go through pictures and magazines with him but also think about using other memorabilia – plane tickets, theater programs, ticket stubs, or party invitations, for example. Of course, if you don't want to use precious originals, make sure to have copies made or even use photocopies or computer printouts.

You can use a store-bought album or simply create a book from individual sheets stapled together. You or your child could create decorative borders around the photos or pictures, or trim around the edges or corners of the photos with one of the many safe corner cutters and scissors on the market that produce scalloped or jagged edges.

Make sure you leave plenty of space to write down the information about the people and places in the pictures, plus any memories that your child wants to record. Ask your child what he wants you to write down about each picture, even if it doesn't seem to make a lot of sense to you. If he wants to, and there is room, you might let him add some drawings to the pages as well.

Add some decorations, too, both to the title page and anywhere else there is room. All children enjoy stickers, so select some that can be used on the front and inside. Ask your child to choose what he wants for each page. While it's generally not recommended to place stickers directly on the photos, let him put them anywhere else on the page that he wants.

KEEP IT SAFE

Closely supervise your child during scrapbooking activities. Provide age-appropriate and nontoxic art materials certified to be safe by the Art & Creative Materials Institute (ACMI). Keep all materials out of reach of young children and teach your youngster how to safely put away all supplies.

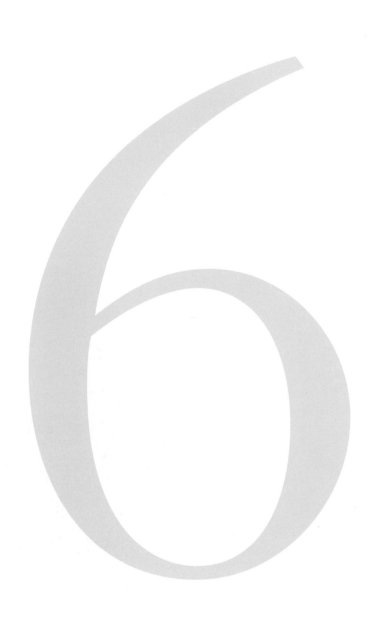
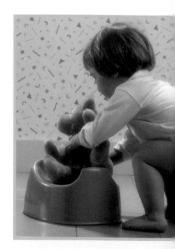

bowel and bladder development

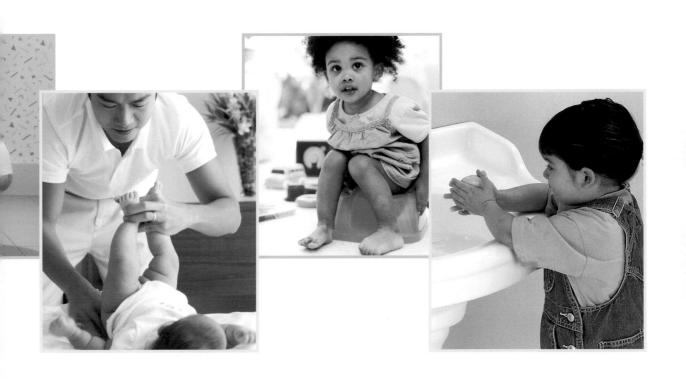

understanding the stages

The achievement of developmental milestones is dependent on the laying down and strengthening of nerve pathways that occurs with increasing age and practice. This is clearly illustrated by the achievement of bowel and bladder control.

At first, the emptying of the bladder and bowel occur as reflex actions that are beyond a child's voluntary control; when stool is present in the lower part of the bowel or a certain volume of urine is present in the bladder, a sequence of events is triggered that leads to a bowel

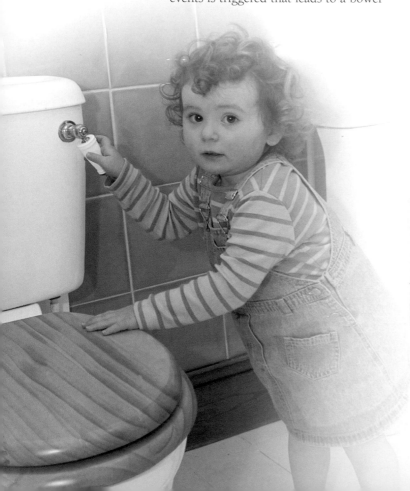

movement or urination. However, as your child matures, additional nerve pathways develop that bring these actions under conscious control. Now a child can learn to resist the urge to urinate or have a bowel movement for a short time, allowing her to reach the potty or toilet. With additional time and practice, a child will learn to control this urge more reliably.

In her own time

Children gain bowel and bladder control when the time is right for them. There is no reason to start toilet training your child before she is ready. If she is not physically mature or emotionally ready, she is not going to be able or motivated to succeed. If any or all of these are the case, wait a while and revisit the situation after a few weeks or months. Most children start to show signs of readiness between 18 months and two and a half years, and bowel and bladder control is generally accomplished at a little over two and a half years of age.

Aiding your child's progress

You can help your child make the transition from diapers to the potty easier by taking the right approach. Being pushy and stressed creates problems, making an issue of something which is, after all, natural. Stay relaxed, be encouraging, and be open about the subject. Children need to be aware that this is a normal part of life and something that everybody has to do.

In addition to talking openly, letting your child accompany you to the toilet may help her understand what is expected of her when she uses the potty. Watching other family members of the same sex is a good way for her to learn about the process. Also, some children like to read stories about using the potty and there are quite a few available on the subject.

It is important to encourage your child to go to the potty or toilet as soon as she needs to. Some children put off going to the toilet, often because they are busy doing something and can't be bothered. This can lead to accidents or constipation and abdominal discomfort.

Try to remain calm and patient even if your child is reluctant to get out of diapers. Don't worry, she will make it sooner or later and having a relaxed approach can only help.

Potty talk

Most children have times when they talk at length about pee and poop. This is completely normal and nothing to worry about. Try not to overreact, it will only make the subject more appealing. Carefully decide what words you use to describe body parts, urine, and bowel movements. It's best to choose simple,

APPROXIMATE TIMING OF EVENTS

The age at which children can begin to be toilet trained varies from child to child. A few may be ready before the age of two years. However, this is relatively uncommon and most will be between two and three when they start to use a potty. Bear in mind that your child, in addition to being able to recognize and control the urge to urinate or defecate, must also be able to remove her clothes quickly and reliably.

From birth:	The bowel and bladder are emptied as a result of a reflex action triggered by the presence of feces and urine. Although babies pass urine and stools at any time, some can, to a certain extent, develop a routine after a few months. They may have a bowel movement after their first morning feeding, for example.
From 2 years:	Your toddler will begin to become aware that her bladder is full and that she needs to urinate. She also becomes aware of the need to pass a bowel movement.
2–4 years:	Many children learn to use a potty successfully around this age. Some of these children become dry at night as soon as they gain bladder and bowel control during the day; for many it takes months or years before night-time diapers can be discarded.
5–6 years:	Most children are dry at night by this age; bed-wetting is usually considered to be a problem after this age. Those who continue to wet the bed after the age of six may do this for a variety of reasons (see also page 177).

proper terms that will not embarrass your child or others.

Hygiene matters

Your child needs to learn about hygiene as soon as she starts using the potty or toilet. However, it is important not to become too obsessive about this because it may lead to her trying to retain bowel movements in order to avoid fuss. Wiping, flushing the toilet, and washing the hands all need to be taught along with using the potty.

You'll need to help your child with wiping until she is about five years old and has the manual dexterity to do it herself.

Flushing upsets some children; they become scared of the noise. Some who use the toilet may worry they may be flushed away. Ask your child what frightens her and then help by showing as best you can her fears are groundless.

PARENTAL PARTICIPATION

Let's pretend

Encourage your child to get familiar with the potty before she uses it. Suggest that she put a stuffed animal or doll on the potty and talk to her about what is happening.

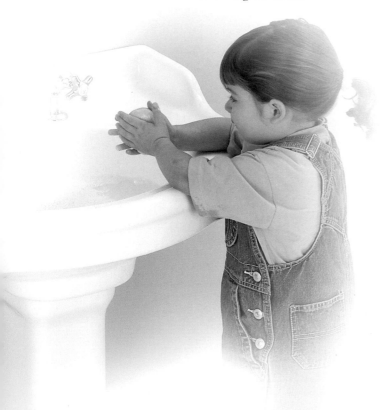

On the other hand, some children really enjoy flushing and, if your child is one of these, you may need to fit a childproof attachment to the handle to prevent her flushing at every opportunity.

Hand-washing should be done after every use of the potty. The best way to teach your child how to do so properly, is to wash your hands at the same time. That way you can show her how to use the soap and how to dry her hands afterward.

Make sure to set your water heater at 120° F or less to prevent your child from burning her hands. Also, as your child gets older teach her to turn on the cold water before the hot.

Position a small stepstool by the sink to make it easier for your child to use.

how the bladder works

The bladder is a muscular sac that stores urine. In young babies it expels urine at intervals as a reflex action. It is only at around two years of age that it begins to be brought under conscious control.

The bladder is made up of four layers of muscle and connective tissue that allow it to expand when it fills with urine. In addition, the bladder has special "stretch receptors" that signal the brain when it needs to be emptied.

Two tubes, the right and left ureters, carry urine from the kidneys to the upper part of the bladder. A larger tube, the urethra, drains urine from the bladder out of the body.

The drainage of urine from the bladder is controlled by two circles of muscle; one, the internal sphincter, lies near the opening to the urethra. It is not under voluntary control. The other, the external sphincter, lies below the internal sphincter and is under voluntary control.

When the volume of urine rises to a specific level, the special stretch receptors in the bladder wall are stimulated. These receptors send messages to the spinal cord, which in turn cause the muscle of the bladder wall to contract. As this reflex is triggered, messages are sent to the brain so we are aware of the need to urinate. The brain also sends messages back to the external sphincter telling it to relax. However, the brain can send messages back to the bladder that ensure that the sphincters remain closed until the time is appropriate to urinate.

Eventually, if the bladder is asked to wait too long to expel its contents, the external sphincter relaxes allowing urine to leak out. An example of this is daytime wetting, which is common in young children because they are often too busy playing to stop and urinate.

In adults and older children, the bladder need not necessarily be full for us to urinate.

What happens in babies

The nerve pathways that send messages from the brain to the bladder do not develop fully until around the age of two years. Prior to this, urination is dependent on the reflex triggered when the volume of urine in the bladder reaches a certain level.

Gaining bladder control

Around the age of two years or more, when the voluntary nerve pathways that connect the brain to the bladder become well developed, a child starts to become aware of needing to urinate and learns to control this urge, by keeping the external sphincter closed until he is able to get to the potty. Interestingly, if a child is denied the chance to use a potty when he first starts to indicate his readiness to be trained, he will probably be late in acquiring full bladder control.

Urinary tract infections in childhood

While these are relatively common in childhood, it is very important to diagnose and treat a suspected urinary tract infection (UTI), because untreated or repeated infections can cause serious illness and long-term medical problems. If you suspect a UTI, contact your pediatrician right away. He or she will examine your child, obtain a urine sample, and prescribe an antibiotic if needed.

Some children may need to be tested for a congenital abnormality in their urinary tract systems, which can predispose them to recurrent UTIs.

Older children tend to complain of the symptoms typical of UTIs in adulthood. These may include pain on passing urine, increased frequency of urination, pain in the abdomen, and, in some cases, blood in the urine. Some older children wet the bed when they have a urinary tract infection. They also may develop a fever. In young children, the symptoms are likely to be more vague and may not necessarily indicate the presence of a urinary tract infection. Like older children, young children may have a fever, but they may also seem unusually fussy or irritable, and eat or drink less. Some may vomit and have diarrhea.

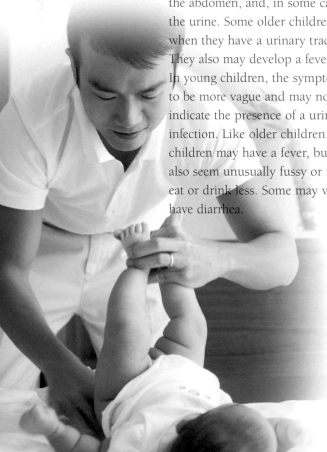

Urgency-frequency syndrome

Also known as Benign Urinary Frequency, this syndrome is a self-limited condition that usually occurs in school-aged children. In this case a toilet-trained child will develop frequent urination during the day. In most cases, the child urinates small amounts, sometimes returning to the bathroom only minutes after finishing. It can last for weeks to months, but eventually goes away on its own. There are no diagnostic tests or treatment, but it is a good idea to see your pediatrician so he or she can make sure a urinary tract infection or other medical problem is not the cause.

Urethritis

Again, a condition that is more commonly seen in girls than boys, urethritis occurs when the opening of the urethra (the tube from which the urine comes out of the bladder) is irritated. This irritation can be caused by bubble bath, soap, or shampoo and is common in school-aged children who spend time playing in the tub. Symptoms include stinging or burning while urinating, feeling the need to urinate frequently or urgently, and itching or pain in the genital area. Since a urinary tract infection can cause similar symptoms, see your pediatrician if your child develops these symptoms. Cleansing the genital area with warm water may relieve any discomfort. To prevent urethritis, avoid bubble bath, reduce exposure to soapy water by washing and shampooing your child at the end of the bath. You could also encourage your child to shower instead.

how the bowel works

The small bowel is where nutrients from food are absorbed into the blood to be processed and used by the body. The large bowel is primarily responsible for getting rid of undigested food and reabsorbing water. Until your child is a toddler, she won't be able to control her bowel movements.

At the end of the large bowel is the rectum; it is 8 inches long in adults, the last 2 inches being the anal canal, which ends in the anus. The anal canal is similar to the outlet of the bladder in that there is an internal anal sphincter, which is not under conscious control, and an external anal sphincter, which is under voluntary control.

Stool can usually remain in the large bowel for as long as a day. The feces are moved along slowly until they reach the rectum. Most of the time, the rectum is empty; once feces enter this final section of the bowel, the urge to pass a bowel movement is experienced. Stretch receptors in the wall of the rectum send messages to the spinal cord, which cause the wall of the lower parts of the bowel to contract and the internal sphincter to relax. The brain also receives messages and if the time is right, it will send messages back to open the external sphincter, allowing feces to pass through. The brain can prevent defecation by causing the external sphincter to remain closed.

Gaining bowel control

Around the age of 18 months to two years, the voluntary nerve pathways that connect the brain to the sphincter become well developed, and a child starts to become aware of needing to pass a bowel movement. Before this time, defecation is uncontrolled, occurring whenever the stretch receptors in the rectum wall trigger the reflex causing the lower large intestine to contract and the internal sphincter to open. Your child learns to control this urge by keeping the external sphincter closed until she is able to get to the potty.

Bowel control is generally acquired before bladder control, as urination is more urgent and immediate. Once bowel control is attained and a child is regularly using the toilet, accidents are usually rare unless there is an emotional problem or an illness that results in loose stools.

Childhood constipation

Like adults, children vary in how often they have a bowel movement. Some will stool once or twice a day; others will stool every few days. Constipation is defined as a decrease in the frequency of bowel movements, the presence of hard stools, and whether your child experiences discomfort on passing a bowel movement.

In some cases, there will be diarrhea when watery feces leak around a hard stool lodged in the bowel.

There are various causes of constipation. Often, it is due to insufficient fluids, perhaps associated with a fever or hot weather or a lack of fiber in the diet. In some cases, problems with toilet training may be a factor.

Sometimes, a child becomes afraid of having a bowel movement. If she has passed a hard stool in the past that has caused pain, for example, she may resist the urge to defecate and hold the stool in. As the feces build up in the lower part of the bowel, fluid continues to be absorbed and the stool gets harder, larger, and more painful to pass. This is a common cycle that causes discomfort and interferes with toilet training. Your child will need treatment to expel the hard stool and then help and advice in learning to return to normal bowel habits.

- -

In the know... *Preventing and treating constipation*
In addition to plenty of water and a healthy diet including lots of fresh vegetables, fruits, and whole grains, the following help to naturally soften your child's stool:
Prune juice, apple juice, pear and apricot nectar
Prunes, plums, grapes, apricots, and cherries
(when age appropriate)
High fiber breads and cereals
Oat bran (added to pancake mix, waffle batter, or oatmeal, for example)

- -

Diarrhea

It is quite common for toddlers to have episodes of loose stools. A loose stool here and there is nothing to worry about, but sudden changes in bowel movements that are much looser and more frequent is considered diarrhea.

Some common causes of diarrhea in toddlers are infection, too much fruit juice, antibiotic use, and toddler's diarrhea. Toddler's diarrhea is a condition that is not fully understood. Children who have it gain weight and grow normally, but have watery, loose stools that often contain pieces of undigested food. The condition is sometimes caused by excessive fluid intake, especially juice and sweetened beverages. Increasing the fat and fiber content in your child's diet and decreasing fluid often will help. Toddler's diarrhea will resolve on its own as your child gets older.

If your child has diarrhea, give her plenty of fluids so she doesn't get dehydrated. Avoid fluids with a high sugar content. Your pediatrician may recommend a pediatric electrolyte solution. Diarrhea also can cause a diaper rash, so apply a zinc oxide diaper cream after every loose bowel movement.

A healthy bowel

All children should have a diet that includes plenty of fluids as well as fruit and vegetables to keep the bowel working well. Whole-grain bread, high-fiber cereals, and dried fruits help to keep the contents of the bowel on the move.

Exercise also plays an important role in keeping the bowel working efficiently. All children should have some form of physical activity every day.

toilet training

As with all developmental achievements, children vary as to when they are ready to learn to use the potty. Between 18 months and two years, children often start to show signs of readiness, but some children may not be ready until two and a half years or older.

Is my child ready?

There are a number of signs that will alert you to when your child may be ready to start using a potty. Some you will notice, others will be brought to your attention!

What you will notice:

* Your child's bowel movements occur on a fairly regular and predictable schedule.
* His diaper is not always wet. Young toddlers urinate often. If diapers remain dry for a couple of hours at a time it suggests that the frequency of urination is slowing.
* Your child is able to follow simple instructions, walk to the bathroom (or potty), and can help undress himself.

What your child may do:

* Get upset when he has a dirty diaper.
* Show signs that he knows that he is about to go in his diaper, such as hiding behind the couch or squatting in a corner.
* Come to tell you or give a sign when he has passed urine or a bowel movement.
* Go and get the potty.
* Sit on the potty – possibly with his diaper on.
* Follow you into the toilet to see what happens.

Making a start

Choose a potty chair that is sturdy and stable. Some children prefer to use an adult sized toilet from the start, in which case it is worth buying a special child-sized seat to fit over your toilet. Your child will also need a stepstool to climb up onto the toilet and to use to push against as his feet won't reach the floor.

Dress your child in clothes that are easy to pull down or hold up. When you

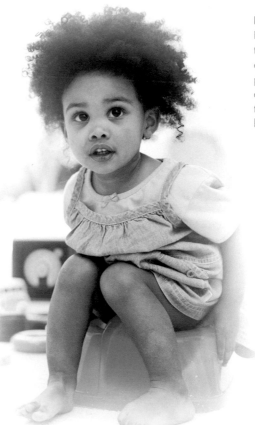

Readiness

For successful potty training, children not only need to be physically aware of any urges to go to the toilet but also need to be emotionally ready.

PARENTAL PARTICIPATION

Share potty chair buying

You can take your child with you when you want to purchase a potty chair. Talk to him about what the potty chair is for.

Make it fun

Don't rush your child when he's on the potty; you can use the time to read some books together and make the experience enjoyable.

Fancy pants

Let your child pick some fun training or underpants that make her feel grown up. Doing so, you can help encourage her to stay dry.

Make it easy

Some children are impatient to start using a regular toilet. A stepstool and special potty seat can make it easier for little ones to reach and use big toilets safely and easily.

Offer praise

Encourage your child with lots of hugs and praise him when success occurs.

can, leave the diaper off – or at least leave his pants off – to give your toddler more chance of getting onto the potty in time. Also remember to:

* **Respond quickly:** If your toddler gives you any sign that he needs to use the potty, lead the way or go and get the potty promptly. Keep in mind that toddlers often become aware that they need to use the potty at the very last minute.

* **Give gentle reminders:** To start with, ask your child every so often whether he wants to go to the potty. When children are busy and having fun they may simply forget. They can have accidents when they are excited, too. Also, remind your child about going to the bathroom when you are going yourself; it will help him if he remembers that this is something everyone needs to do.

As toddlers get older, they may resist frequent reminders, so try to support your child's urge to be independent as much as possible.

* *Stick to your child's schedule:* Some toddlers urinate and have bowel movements at particular times during the day. If this applies to your child, encourage him to use the potty at these times.

* *Encourage your child:* Give him plenty of praise when he manages to tell you he needs to use the potty or goes to it himself.

* *Be calm when accidents happen:* Accidents are inevitable in the early days. Clean up your child and change his clothes right away, saying that it was an accident. It also helps to involve your child in the cleanup.

* *And remember to be patient and positive:* It may take some time for your child to use the potty reliably and he will have setbacks along the way. Stay confident, offer praise, and be encouraging.

Is there a problem?

If you aren't getting anywhere when you first begin, don't worry; it probably means that your child is not ready for toilet training yet. Go back to using diapers and stop talking about the potty-training process. Leave the potty in an easily accessible place for when he decides to return to it.

In few cases, however, there may be a specific underlying cause for the problem. Possible causes include:

* *Are you pushing your child?:* Take a step back and relax. Putting a child under pressure will be counterproductive and make him resist the potty.

* *Is your child under stress?:* Disruptions or changes at home or at child care can be a cause. These also can cause a child to wet during the day when he was previously dry.

* *Does he need more reminders?:* Remember to keep them gentle and casual.

* *Is he getting enough sleep?:* Toddlers can have problems with getting to the potty at the right time if they are overtired.

* *Is there a physical cause?:* This is relatively uncommon and a urinary tract infection is the most common. If your child continues to wet without an obvious cause or if he seems to urinate frequently, finds urination painful, or passes blood in the urine, see your pediatrician. You should also call your pediatrician if your child starts to have accidents again after a period of dryness. Your pediatrician may run some simple tests, like testing a sample of urine to look for an infection.

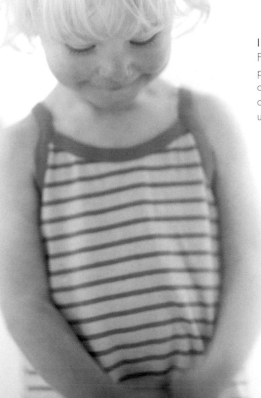

I have to go
Facial expressions, posture, or words are all signs that your child may need to use the potty.

becoming dry at night

Bed-wetting is extremely common and is not usually considered to be a problem until a child is six years or older. Children vary in the age they achieve nighttime dryness. For most, it is a natural progression from being dry during the day; for others, it may be years before they become dry at night. By five or six years of age, most children are dry at night.

With young children it is important to let nature take its course; don't push your child by saying that she should be wearing underpants at night or during nap times.

A good time to try her in underpants is when your child still has a dry diaper on waking and is ready to stop wearing diapers at night. However, it may help to put a plastic sheet or other waterproof bedcover under the sheet for some time in case accidents occur.

When you first make the transition, don't be disappointed if your child wets the bed – just change the bedding and let her know it's not her fault. It helps to involve your child in the process.

If your child is wetting the bed every night, suggest she goes back into diapers or training pants for a while and try again after a few weeks. There is no point in continuing if she is not having success – this is just upsetting for both of you.

Is my child ready?

Here are some of the signs that your child may be getting ready to stop wearing diapers or training pants at night:
* She is dry in the morning.
* She gets up in the night to urinate.
* She comes to tell you that her diaper is wet.
* She tells you she wants to start wearing underpants.

Helping your child stay dry at night
* *Limit fluids:* Avoid drinking large amounts of fluid before bedtime.
* *Lifting:* You may try taking your child

PARENTAL PARTICIPATION

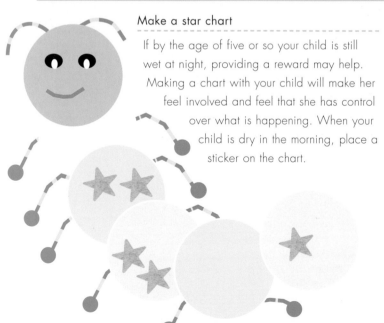

Make a star chart

If by the age of five or so your child is still wet at night, providing a reward may help. Making a chart with your child will make her feel involved and feel that she has control over what is happening. When your child is dry in the morning, place a sticker on the chart.

to the toilet when you go to bed and possibly if you happen to get up in the night. However, it is not worth doing this if it disrupts your child's sleep and makes her tired during the day.

* **Last visit:** Make sure your child urinates just before she goes to bed. Encourage her to use the toilet even if she doesn't want to by incorporating it into her bedtime routine.

* **Using thinner diapers:** Often, thick diapers or really absorbent training pants that really do their job will feel dry on the inside when a child has urinated. This may hamper a child from learning about the sensation of needing to get up and urinate. Wearing a thinner diaper that becomes a little damp on the inside may help.

* **Keep calm:** Some children take longer than others to achieve nighttime dryness. Because you want your child to do this naturally, stay relaxed when accidents happen. Never punish your child for being wet at night! Your pediatrician will be able to offer help and advice.

* **Give praise:** Although you don't want to make a fuss when things go wrong, it is equally important to praise your child when she manages to stay dry.

Is there a problem?

In most cases, delayed nighttime dryness indicates that a child is just not ready to be dry. Other reasons for bed-wetting have been suggested, such as having a small bladder, but not all of the causes are fully understood. However, we do know that bed-wetting and late achievement of nighttime dryness seem to run in the family – if either parent was late in doing this, there is a good chance that their child

will be, too. Bed-wetting is also more common in boys – the reason for this is not known.

If your child is still having problems staying dry at night after the age of five, talk to your pediatrician not only to exclude an underlying medical problem but also for some advice on how to manage the issue.

Enuresis (bed-wetting) alarms

These may be recommended from the age of six. Urinating in the night sets the alarm buzzer off which wakes the child. The aim is that she will eventually become aware of when she needs to urinate and will get up herself.

7

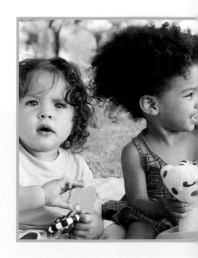

developmental concerns

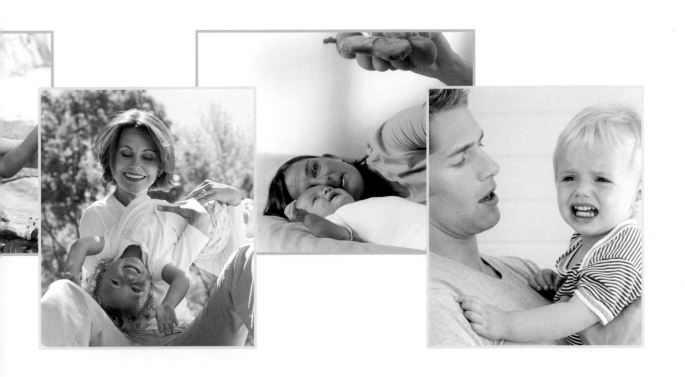

DEVELOPMENTAL CONCERNS

In this chapter you can read about some common developmental concerns such as late walking, delayed speech, and hyperactivity, and learn to distinguish between a condition, which may hold your child back, and delay, which will improve over time or require intervention services. Bear in mind that delay in reaching a milestone can run in families, and is much more common than a medical cause.

Many parents worry about their child's development and how that will affect him at school and in social situations. Even an overly bright child can be challenging. An attentive dad or mom is the best person to tell if his or her child is developing normally. If you have any specific concerns, don't be afraid to let your pediatrician know. Be sure to trust your own judgment but do remember that every baby and toddler is different and they all may develop at their own rate. The most important thing with many childhood developmental conditions is that they are detected early, and that parents understand the circumstances and are provided with extra support or services early on in order to help their child.

Developmental delay

The preceding six chapters covered the normal stages of acquiring movement, fine motor, sensory, mental, and social skills as well as bowel and bladder control. Delay occurs when the milestones are not met within the expected range of normal. However, there is a wide range for which many milestones will be achieved and many children will ultimately develop normally despite having a delay in reaching a specific milestone.

Developmental delay is most commonly discussed in terms of independent sitting, walking, and speaking, and the main reasons for such delay will be covered under the appropriate topics below. But there are other kinds of delay, too, which perceptive parents may notice. For example: Delay in fixing or following an object with the eyes, in holding the head up, in smiling, in reaching out or exchanging an item from hand to hand, and in rolling. The first of these is discussed later in this chapter under sensory impairment. With the others, the usual advice would be to ask the advice of your child's pediatrician.

Delay in unsupported sitting

A baby will generally sit unsupported between six to eight months of age. The most common reasons for not doing so are:
* Prematurity (a baby who is two months premature is likely to sit two months later than a baby born on time);
* Not provided with enough opportunities to sit;
* Familial factors, e.g. parents were late walkers;
* Medical conditions such as cerebral palsy or muscular weakness;
* Global developmental delay.
The last two are the most serious. Cerebral palsy is thought to be caused by malformation or damage

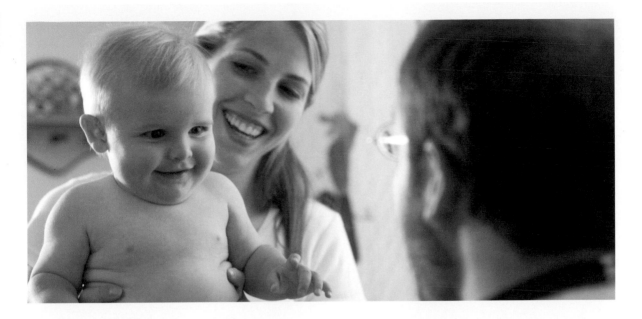

to the developing brain during pregnancy, delivery, or immediately after birth. The condition causes different types of challenges, including motor disability, which can vary from mild to severe. Intelligence may be normal, but associated cognitive or learning problems frequently do occur. Many programs and special services are available to help children with cerebral palsy, including physical and occupational therapy.

Global developmental delay means a delay in all the milestones and may be due to a congenital disorder of the brain or underlying syndrome or disease. In some cases no cause can be found despite extensive testing.

If your child doesn't appear to be anxious to sit, let your pediatrician know so he or she can examine your child for an increase or decrease in muscle tone.

You can help your child yourself by encouraging him to sit and propping him up. You also can encourage muscle use in other ways such as spending time on the floor with him and allowing him to push up, roll, crawl, and reach out for toys.

Talk it through
As parents, you are in the best position to know whether your child is developing normally. However, if you have any specific concerns about your child's development, talk to your pediatrician.

Delay in walking

Walking requires very great skill, coordination, and confidence, so that a baby's personality and environment play a role in when and how he goes about this. As well as the factors described above for delayed sitting, the excessive use of a stationary baby walker may delay independent walking (see page 32). In addition, there are many medical conditions, such as cerebral palsy, global developmental delay, and muscular dystrophy, that interfere with walking.

Muscular dystrophy (MD) is a rare muscle disease that leads to progressive weakness. It usually occurs in boys. One cause of late walking is due to muscle weakness. If your child is not walking independently by 16 to 18 months, talk to your pediatrician.

Hypotonia

Hypotonia is a term used to describe low muscle tone and as such it is a description of a clinical finding and not a diagnosis of a disease or disorder.

A child with low tone has muscles that are slow to begin a muscle contraction, contract very slowly in response to a stimulus, and cannot maintain a contraction for as long as other children. Children with hypotonia are sometimes described as "floppy" because they have the look and feel of a rag doll. They are not able to maintain any position for very long, such as holding their heads up or holding out their arms. In the severe form, there may be difficulties with feeding and with moving around.

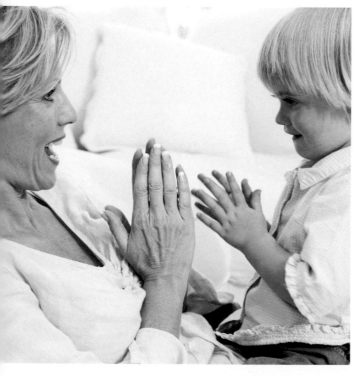

What may cause hypotonia?

Although hypotonia is associated with conditions such as Down syndrome, cerebral palsy, and muscular dystrophy, it also can occur in otherwise normal, healthy infants. In these cases, the babies may be somewhat delayed in the motor milestones. They are prone to walking late and may shuffle or scoot for a longer than usual time.

Testing understanding
It's not hard to make sure your child has some idea of what is going on around her. Although she may not be able to answer any questions, you can ask her to do something – like clapping her hands or handing you a toy – and she should respond correctly.

How to help a child with hypotonia

If you are concerned about your child being hypotonic or floppy, then consult your pediatrician. Further testing may be necessary.

If the hypotonia is more severe, there is a range of tests that may be considered. Physical therapy may be of benefit. Helping your child to develop her muscles through appropriate activity is always valuable.

Delay in speech and language development

The acquisition of words can be set back by a number of factors. The most important reasons a child doesn't speak are that he is not spoken to or that he has a hearing loss (see page 186). Sometimes a child who has older siblings finds that they anticipate his every need, and take away one of the normal stimuli for learning new words. For example, they may answer questions for him or give him exactly what he wants when he points to it.

Another is when a child has temporary impairment of hearing due to chronic fluid behind the ear drum that accumulates because of one or more colds. This muffles the hearing and makes it very difficult for a child to learn new words. Other reasons include global delay and specific medical or language disorders, such as autism.

Even before you expect your child to speak, you should check that he is beginning to understand what you say and uses gestures such as waving, pointing, and clapping by nine to 12 months. Some children seem to understand a lot but not speak much until they are over two years old, so it is very important to check out your child's understanding and gestures. Can he point to parts of the body? (Around 18 months.) Will he get his shoes from the bedroom when you ask? (Around 16 months.) Does

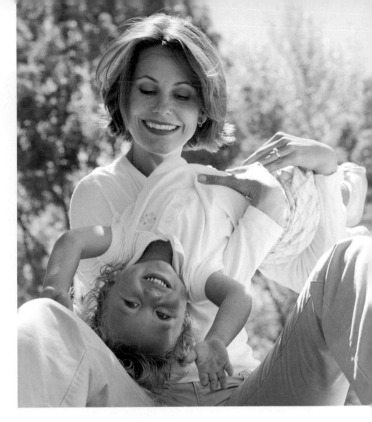

Muscle building exercise
Activity is important to building muscle tone in both normal children and those affected by hypotonia.

he wave when you say "bye-bye?" (Around nine months.) Does he point to objects? (Around 12 months.) If his understanding seems behind, speak to your pediatrician. In some cases, referral to a speech therapist or another professional may be needed.

Hearing should always be tested as your child may hear normally at some frequencies but not at the ones needed for speech discrimination.

The most important things for children with speech delay is to expose them to language often. Don't push your child into talking, but talk to him as often as possible by describing what is going on and making it fun. Read your child books and use stories and pictures to describe events and point to colors, animals, and activities when you are out.

Often, professionals such as speech therapists can help, and your pediatrician can make a referral, if necessary.

Sensory impairment

The five senses are hearing, vision, smell, taste, and touch. While hearing and vision are both central to the abilities and achievement of a human being and important for communication, there are many individuals who have overcome their disability in these fields to achieve success in their lives. Early detection and treatment is important.

Hearing impairment

Hearing loss is the most common congenital abnormality in the USA – about 12,000 babies are born annually with hearing loss. Hearing is essential to speech and language development. Babies who do not hear well will not develop normal speech or will develop it late. All newborns should undergo a screening test shortly after birth in the hospital and this should accurately detect babies with severe congenital hearing loss. This can be caused by:
* Congenital infection (infection occurring before birth), e.g. Rubella (German measles), CMV (cytomegalovirus);
* Malformation of the ear;
* Drugs taken during pregnancy;
* Prematurity;
* Genetic conditions.

However, a hearing impairment may be acquired after birth from the following causes:
* Head injury or ear trauma;
* Severe infection (e.g. meningitis);
* Certain medications.

Parents will notice quite early if their infant does not hear by the following signs. The baby doesn't:
* Startle when there is a loud noise (from birth);
* Turn her head to a nearby noise or music (by five months);
* Develop the usual infant babble (around six months) or babbling decreases instead of progressing.

Hearing loss affecting the inner ear is described as sensorineural, and that affecting the middle ear is called conductive hearing loss.

Effects of hearing loss

Hearing loss or hearing impairment ranges from mild to very severe and may affect one or both ears. Some children have no hearing at all, and they will take longer to develop language. Hearing impairment may also be limited to only part of the sound range, e.g. the high tones. This type may be hard to detect as the child has some hearing, but because he cannot hear words clearly, his speech may be markedly delayed.

If your child has only partial hearing loss, you may not be aware of this until it is apparent that his speech is delayed. If you suspect hearing loss, always consult your pediatrician. Your child may be referred to an audiologist or an ear, nose, and throat specialist, who will carry out further tests.

Helping a child with a hearing impairment

Nowadays, there is a wide range of services available in addition to hearing aids. Hearing aids are much smaller, more effective, and harder to discern than previously. While a hearing aid may restore hearing to normal or near-normal levels in a child with conductive hearing loss, it will not restore hearing completely to a child with significant sensorineural hearing loss. A cochlear implant may be recommended for children 12 months of age or older who have profound hearing loss in both ears, and who receive little or no benefit from hearing aids. This is a surgically implanted device that sends sound information via electrical stimulation directly to the auditory nerve, bypassing the damaged, missing, or nonfunctioning sensory receptors located within the inner ear.

Speech therapists can help a child with sensorineural hearing loss to lip-read, use sign language, and speak. Specialists in sign language can teach you and your child to sign. Some children learn to lip-read well. At school, your child should be able to have access to educational support and specialized teachers.

Visual impairment

Visual impairment varies from a child with severe visual acuity problems to a child who has very little vision, the majority being at the milder end of the spectrum. Visual impairment may be detected at birth or soon after. During the routine newborn exams, your pediatrician will check your infant's eyes for signs of structural defects, cataracts, or glaucoma, as well as that your baby fixes on your eyes and, in later months, follows an object around the room. Within the first few weeks of their expected date of delivery, babies should be able to fix and follow an interesting object either side of the midline. If needed, more sophisticated tests can distinguish whether there is a delay in maturation, with no other consequences, or whether something more serious is the problem.

However like hearing impairment, a milder visual impairment will only be detected by specialized testing. Since problems with vision can appear at any time in childhood, your pediatrician will check your child's eyes during all routine well-child exams.

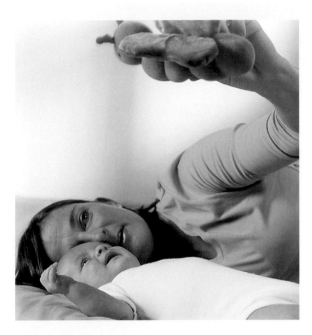

Hearing check
Parents are a child's first line in assessing abilities. If her hearing is normal, your young baby should turn toward the direction of a persistent sound.

Causes of visual impairment

There are a multitude of types and causes but the common ones are:

* Strabismus. This is a misalignment of the eyes caused by an imbalance or weakness of the muscles that control the eye. If not detected early or left untreated, it can damage vision;

* Amblyopia. This condition is sometimes referred to as "lazy eye." It occurs when the brain and the eye aren't working together properly, usually because the eye itself is weak or injured, causing misalignment of the eyes. Can also be caused by strabismus. Early detection and treatment is important to preserve a child's vision;

* The structure of the eye or of the visual pathways is abnormal from birth: e.g. coloboma, a gap or cleft in one of the structures of the eye;

* The vision system is damaged by an illness, cerebral palsy, or condition of prematurity;
* The vision system may be normal or appear normal structurally at birth but lose sight either quickly or slowly due to degeneration;
* A preterm baby may suffer from retinopathy of prematurity, especially if he required oxygen over a prolonged period.

The child who is visually impaired will rely very much on hearing for communication. As always, early diagnosis and treatment is critical for a child to develop and learn to his full potential.

If you suspect any problems with vision, consult your pediatrician. He or she may recommend an ophthalmologist, who will carry out tests to diagnose the cause of the condition, assess the degree of visual impairment, and discuss available treatment options. Specialized teaching support services will ensure that the child's educational needs are met.

The eyes are often suspected of being implicated in learning problems, but are almost never the cause. Even with dyslexia, it is the brain's processing of stimuli that causes difficulties, not a visual problem.

Language delays

Language is central to our ability to function as human beings. To communicate effectively we need language. Speech is only one part of language and before children can speak, they need to hear and understand what other people are saying, they need to process the language, and they need to formulate the concepts. Unfortunately, there are many possible problems, which may develop so that the child's speech is not well understood.

Language impairment refers to the particular difficulties that some children may suffer as a result of a problem with language. Among these children are those who:

* Have reasonable comprehension, but are unable to express themselves appropriately;
* Have limited understanding of spoken language.

Stuttering

Stuttering is common (more so in boys than girls), tends to run in families, and is a considerable cause of concern for parents. It normally appears between the ages of two and five, and for many children will resolve on its own by the time they enter school. The child who stutters may repeat a word or part of a word and may show a particular facial expression when trying to speak.

As with all the problems outlined here, discuss the issue with your pediatrician. He or she may refer your child to a speech and language therapist.

POSITIVE PARENTING

There is a lot you can do to help if your child stutters.

Don't ask your child to:
- slow down;
- repeat the word;
- think before he speaks.

Do:
- listen carefully to your child, concentrating on the meaning not the fluency;
- slow down your own rate of talking; don't ask too many questions;
- allow him to finish, you shouldn't finish the sentence for him;
- praise what is done well to increase confidence.

Articulation problems

This group of disorders affect a child's ability to develop easily understood speech. Some children with articulation disorders also have language difficulties such as immature grammar and syntax, stuttering, or word-retrieval difficulties that can affect their abilities to learn to read or spell.

Many children may use incorrect consonants (e.g. car becomes tar), or omit one of the two or three consonants that occur together in a word (e.g. bread sounds like bed). As a result, the words may be understandable by parents more so than strangers, which may sometimes lead to frustration and embarrassment.

Articulation problems may be due to immaturity; poor control of the lip, tongue, and palate muscles used for speech; because the family understands the child anyway; or to recurrent middle ear infections, which affect a child's ability to hear differences among similar sounds.

Children with articulation problems do not necessarily go on to experience literacy problems, and most have no difficulty learning to read and spell. It is important to seek treatment when you first notice your child may be having difficulty.

Not all children will require therapy; some need a little extra time to catch up with their peers. Again, talk to your pediatrician if you are concerned about your child's speech, as early speech therapy intervention may be of benefit.

Frustration
It's normal for a toddler to become angry or frustrated when he can't make himself understood. By age 2, at least 50 percent of what he says should be understandable to a stranger, 75 percent by age 3, and 100 percent by age 4.

Disruptive behavior

Virtually all children go through disruptive phases. Disruptiveness is related to temperament, parenting style, and environment. Many, but not all, children tend to fall into one of three broad and loosely defined categories: easy, slow to warm up or shy, or difficult or challenging. These labels are a useful shorthand, but none can offer a complete picture of a child. Many parents find it more useful to think about their child in terms of nine temperamental traits.

✳ *Activity level:* How much physical activity, restlessness, or fidgety behavior a child demonstrates in daily activities (and which also may affect sleep).

✳ *Rhythmicity or regularity:* The presence or absence of a regular pattern for basic physical functions such as appetite, sleep, and bowel habits.

✳ *Approach and withdrawal:* The way a child initially responds to a new stimulus (rapid and bold

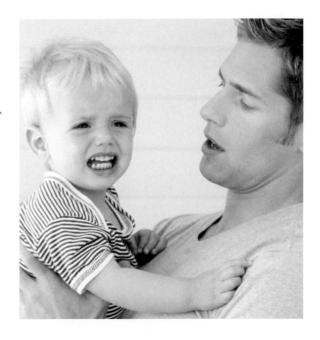

or slow and hesitant), whether it be people, situations, places, foods, or changes in routines.

* *Adaptability:* The degree of ease or difficulty with which a child adjusts to change or a new situation, and how well the youngster can modify his reaction.

* *Intensity:* The energy level with which a child responds to a situation, whether positive or negative.

* *Mood:* The degree of pleasantness or unfriendliness in a child's words and behavior.

* *Attention span:* The ability to concentrate or stay with a task, with or without distraction.

* *Distractibility:* The ease with which a child can be distracted from a task by environmental (usually visual or auditory) stimuli.

* *Sensory threshold:* The amount of stimulation needed for a child to respond. Some children respond to the slightest stimulation, others require more.

Consistency is very important for children, both in respect to their daily routine and discipline, and support and involvement in their activities. In addition, providing your children with plenty of encouragement will help foster a positive environment both in the home and away. When parents are inconsistent with discipline, are not supportive and positive, and do not participate in their child's activities, it will negatively affect a child's behavior. Watching aggressive behavior on TV or in videos, or participation in aggressive games will only encourage your child to become more disruptive.

Managing disruptive behaviors in a preschool child

Temperamental characteristics associated with disruptive behavior include aggression, attention-seeking, and lack of empathy.

Children who are at the preverbal level will communicate through their behavior as they are unable to put their feelings into words. So if your child is being disruptive, this is likely to be the result of his feelings: anger, fear, anxiety, or frustration. You can defuse the situation by commenting on the emotion rather than on the behavior. To parent such a child successfully, you should try and understand the situation and predict in advance when fireworks may arise. In general, if you treat your child as described in the Positive Parenting box, disruptive behavior should decrease.

POSITIVE PARENTING

There are many things you can do to manage a temperamentally difficult child:

* Keep your child active, with plenty of outdoor activities;
* Praise her whenever she is being calm and helpful, or playing quietly;
* Give her reasonable special time each day when she can choose the activity;
* Make sure that she knows the rules about relationships, e.g. politeness and consideration (not easy for a preschool child); teaching problem-solving skills can never start too young;
* Explain in advance what will happen if she is disruptive (does she know what this means?);
* Ignore behavior that is boisterous and energetic but not hurtful or harmful;
* Set a limit on media activities;
* Set rules for "unacceptable" behavior – e.g. fighting, hurting a sibling, or damaging toys;
* Use time-out if she oversteps the limits (see right.)

Time-out

This is a procedure that can be used for any young child as part of a strategy to improve his behavior. It involves sending your child to a specified place, such as a chair, with no entertaining distractions (not his bedroom, for example) for a set period of time – generally one minute for each year of age. Before using time-out, you need to explain that you will tell your child what he needs to do or stop doing to avoid the time-out and that you will give him a warning before you institute it so that he has a chance to change his behavior. Time-out needs to be used in conjunction with positive reinforcement of desired behaviors and only should be used when your child understands the reason; it should not be used for nonspecific "bad behavior."

Managing disruptive behaviors in a school-age child

Disruptiveness in an older child is harder to deal with because the poor behavior lasts longer and may occur in school as well. What makes older children disruptive? Common reasons are:

* Difficulties with school work, perhaps due to learning difficulties;

* Bullying at school;

* Undiagnosed and untreated ADHD or autistic spectrum disorder;

* Insufficient emotional support and quality time with parents;

* Lack of adequate boundary setting at home;

* Parental conflict or change in the family structure.

A disruptive school-age child may be very stressful for parents if the difficulties show up in school as well as at home. If your child is disruptive, it is important to maintain close relationships with the principal and key teachers. Bullying is frequently a factor and can be very distressing. Children do not

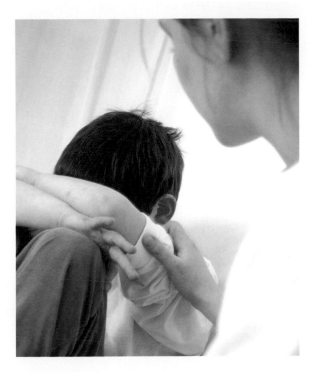

Effective discipline
A good relationship, praise, and instructing your child on how to control his behavior is the key to both encouraging good habits and changing negative ones.

always like to admit to being bullied, so you may need to tease out the information.

If you find things are getting out of control, or as soon as symptoms are noticed, consult your pediatrician, who will be able to talk to your child separately and also look for other factors that may be influencing the behavior.

ADHD

Attention Deficit Hyperactivity Disorder (ADHD) causes problems with inattention and/or hyperactivity and impulsivity that are inappropriate for your child's developmental level and are impairing your child's performance across settings. ADHD is seen in three common types:

* Inattentive only:
Children with this type (formerly known as ADD) are not overly active. They do not disrupt the classroom or other activities, so their symptoms may not be noticed. This is the most common form found in girls.

* Hyperactive/impulsive:
Children with this type of ADHD show both hyperactive and impulsive behavior, but are able to pay attention.

* Combined inattentive/hyperactive/impulsive:
Children with this type show all three symptoms; this is the most common type.

SYMPTOMS OF ADHD

SYMPTOM	BEHAVIOR
Inattention:	Has a hard time paying attention, daydreams.
	Does not seem to listen.
	Is easily distracted from work or play.
	Does not seem to care about details, makes careless mistakes.
	Does not follow through on instructions or finish tasks.
	Is disorganized.
	Loses a lot of important things.
	Forgets things.
	Does not want to do things that require ongoing mental effort.
Hyperactivity:	Is in constant motion, as if "driven by a motor."
	Cannot stay seated.
	Squirms and fidgets.
	Talks too much.
	Runs, jumps, and climbs when this is not permitted.
	Cannot play quietly.
Impulsivity:	Acts and speaks without thinking.
	May run into the street without looking for traffic first.
	Has trouble taking turns.
	Cannot wait for things.
	Calls out answers before the question is complete.
	Interrupts others.

ADHD means what it says: a child who is on the go all the time, who has difficulty in concentrating, and who is impulsive (does things without thinking). Since most preschool children normally show these symptoms, the diagnosis is not usually made before the age of six. There is no specific test to diagnose ADHD. It occurs in 4 to 12 percent of the population and is more common in boys. ADHD may cause difficulty for both parents and teachers, and if untreated, can significantly affect learning and progress in school and social interactions with peers. So it is important to get help if you think your child has ADHD.

ADHD is one of the most common chronic conditions of childhood. It is a biological disorder. It can be diagnosed by appropriate clinical assessment and then treated. Often, medication can help ADHD symptoms at school, home, and in their other activities. In addition to medication, behavior therapy, education, parent training, and counseling are all important in helping a child with ADHD succeed.

Since it is very common for children to exhibit behavioral problems, how is the diagnosis of ADHD made? As there is no biochemical test, parents, teachers, and other caregivers are relied upon to provide evidence of the core symptoms – developmentally inappropriate levels of inattention, impulsivity, hyperactivity – the duration the symptoms have been noticed, and an assessment of the degree to which they interfere with their child's ability to function. And, as the child will generally be of school age, the pediatrician also will ask for information from the child's teacher or other school professional. Special checklists exist and often are used to identify the key symptoms.

If you suspect that your child has ADHD, you should consult your pediatrician. It is usually

CONFIRMING A DIAGNOSIS OF ADHD

The behaviors in the chart on page 192, must:

- Occur in more than one setting, such as home, school, and social situations;
- Be more severe than in other children the same developmental age;
- Start before the child reaches 7 years of age. (However, these may not be recognized as ADHD symptoms until a child is older);
- Continue for more than 6 months;
- Make it difficult to function at school, at home, and/or in social situations.

beneficial for more than one professional to be involved in the diagnosis, and a report from the school should be obtained. Your pediatrician may use a checklist to collect information from home and school, as well as taking a careful history.

Once a diagnosis is made, management will be discussed. The modes of treatment are medication, behavior therapy, and support in school. Your pediatrician should also check if there are other conditions present such as learning disabilities (such as dyslexia), or symptoms of anxiety, depression, or oppositional and conduct problems.

Medication

If your child is diagnosed with ADHD, medication can improve ADHD symptoms. It can help a child focus her thoughts better and ignore distractions. This will enable her to pay more attention and to control her behavior, improving her school performance and ability to succeed in social activities. The medications most commonly prescribed are stimulants. These help to focus attention, control impulses, organize and plan, and stick to routines. They are prescribed in a variety of doses and schedules. Some children respond to one type of stimulant but not another. In addition, there are several nonstimulant medications to treat ADHD. It may take some time to find the best medication, dose, and schedule for your child. Your pediatrician or child psychiatrist will follow your child closely and adjust the medication as needed.

Behavior therapy

In addition to medication, parents can be taught to manage and shape their child's behavior so as to encourage the positive aspects and control the

negative. By doing so, family interactions can be improved and the child can better manage her own behavior. Parents can be provided with a set of practical, tested procedures that can help them respond appropriately to different situations – providing either praise or punishment or ignoring the behavior. Many of the techniques are those set out in the Positive Parenting box on page 190.

Support in school

A child with ADHD may need extra support in school. Be sure to talk to the principal and teacher about your child's condition, so that everyone can work together to ensure that your child succeeds in the classroom. Management techniques that work well for children with ADHD include:

* Keeping a set routine and schedule for activities;

* Using a system of clear rewards and consequences;

Plays well with others
Engaging with others and making a sociable companion are signs that your child is developing a rounded personality.

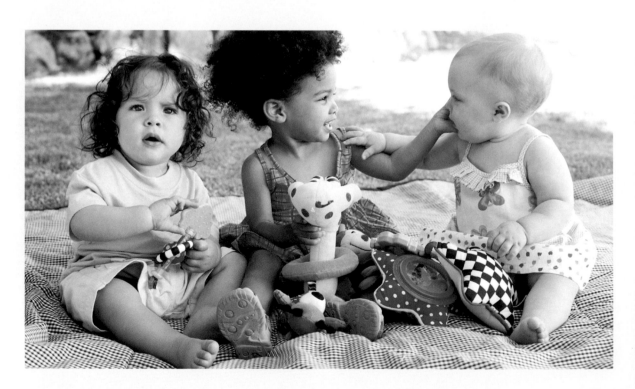

* Sending daily or weekly report cards or behavior charts to parents;
* Seating the child near the teacher;
* Using small groups for activities;
* Encouraging students to pause a moment before answering questions;
* Keeping assignments short or breaking them into sections;
* Close supervision with frequent, positive cues to stay on task.

Remember that once diagnosed and treated, children with ADHD, are more likely to achieve their goals in school and succeed in life.

Autism Spectrum Disorders (ASDs)

Autism is the name given to a condition that causes a disability in social interactions. A child with an autistic disorder has three characteristics: he doesn't communicate well, both verbally and nonverbally; he has atypical social skills; and his behavior is often repetitive and obsessional. However, autism can be difficult to diagnose because the range of severity is quite wide, so professionals often talk of the autism spectrum.

Autism is a complex disorder with symptoms that range from mild to severe. There is a big difference between children with classical autism and those with Asperger syndrome; the latter children will demonstrate significant social deficits but also will have well-developed verbal skills, despite a significant deficit in communicating socially.

Like ADHD, autism is much more common in boys than girls. A child with core autism will have the features as detailed in the box above.

Children with autism do not make the usual eye contact or use facial expressions in social situations.

FEATURES OF CLASSICAL AUTISM

- Delayed, absent, or atypical expressive speech and understanding; the child may not speak any words before two years of age;
- Lack of joint attention (lack of eye contact, response to name, pointing, showing toys/objects to others);
- Lack of emotional engagement — doesn't like kisses and cuddles;
- Prefers to play alone, often for long periods;
- Lack of imaginative play — often lines up cars or spends long periods looking at curtains or light;
- Repetitive behavior, e.g. rocking or spinning;
- Difficult behavior is common;
- All milestones may be delayed; but language and social skills are often more delayed than nonverbal, visual problem-solving, and motor skills.

They are less likely to use gestures such as pointing to communicate. They tend to find it difficult to cooperate, share, or take turns. They prefer to play alone, and show no interest in imaginative play. They tend to get along best with understanding adults. Socializing with other children and forming friendships is hard for them. These features are quite distinctive. If your child displays any of these symptoms, consult your pediatrician. However, the autistic spectrum is broad and much milder degrees may be present.

The features of Asperger syndrome, which is at the milder end of the autism spectrum, are shown in the box on page 196. Some signs for parents to watch for are social isolation, lack of emotional rapport, and dislike of changes in routine.

FEATURES OF ASPERGER SYNDROME

- Rigidity of thinking;
- Dislike of changes in routine;
- Poor social skills;
- Poor understanding of emotions;
- Very good memory of events and facts;
- Often considerable interest and talent in a particular field;
- May talk at length about her interest, without showing reciprocal interest;
- Difficulty at school because of nonverbal communication and social skills deficits;
- Behavioral problems due to the above;
- Often picked on and bullied at school.

routine, explain instructions carefully to be sure that their child understands what is being requested, and help their child to develop social skills. It is also important to obtain extra support in school. The earlier the intervention is started, the better, so consult your pediatrician if you have any concerns about your child.

Because parenting a child with ASD is usually stressful, family support is often considered a vital part of an overall intervention plan. Families with more support from other parents and community organizations have less stress. Trained individuals, known as respite services, may be available to look after a child with ASD when extended family or friends are not available.

Who can provide help?

If you think that your child might have an autistic spectrum disorder, consult your pediatrician. Because it is a complex disorder, a comprehensive evaluation is required along with a neurological assessment and cognitive and language testing. As with other children with speech delay, children suspected of autism should have their hearing evaluated by a pediatric audiologist.

A multidisciplinary team, including your pediatrician, a neurologist, developmental pediatrician or psychiatrist, psychologist, speech therapist, and other professionals, can help diagnose and treat autism.

There is no cure for autism, but early, intensive behavioral intervention can improve specific symptoms and bring about substantial improvement.

There is very much that can be done to help a child with autism. Parents need to maintain a

POSITIVE PARENTING

Children with ASD require intensive early intervention services from health professionals. There are also things you can do to help your child with ASD.

- Join in your child's activities. Talk with your child about what he is playing with and what he is doing with it. Try and keep a back-and-forth interaction going;
- Point at interesting objects and reward your child with praise when he makes the appropriate responses;
- Teach your child to point at things that he wants or things that interest him instead of crying or leading you by the hand. Make sure to acknowledge it when he shows you something of interest to him.

Gifted children

The term "gifted" and "talented" is used within educational circles to describe children with ability levels above the average. Usually, parents will notice that their child is more advanced than other children of a comparable age. The child will reach milestones more quickly, particularly in the fields of language development and literacy, mathematics, music, or athletics. She is likely to be a good reader early, show an aptitude and interest in study, be imaginative, and will have advanced abstract thinking.

Sometimes a child is not detected as being gifted until starting school. The high level of ability is not always recognized initially, and the child may become bored and display behavioral difficulties because the level of work is too simple.

If you think that your child might have unusual talents, then it would be very important to discuss this with the teacher or principal as it is important to pick this up early.

Management of gifted children

Parents of a gifted child should take professional advice from teachers and other specialists on how to handle their child. Most advisers caution against advancing a child too fast with the aim of developing a genius.

A normal childhood is a requirement for all children and it will be of no benefit to your child to be placed in a high pressure environment. On the other hand, teaching should be sufficient to challenge your child and allow her to progress at a pace that suits her rather than the average child of the same age.

Being a good parent to a gifted child often involves a lot of energy to keep up with her many interests. Because she is still only a child, albeit a very bright one, you need to ensure that she is not overstimulated and that her creative juices are allowed to flow through play of all types. You also need to ensure that you manage the other aspects of her development.

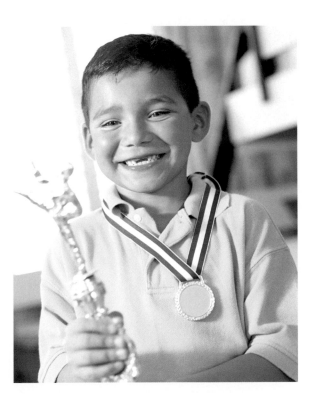

Bright but balanced
The challenge of parenting a gifted child is to make sure that other aspects of his development – social, emotional, and spiritual, for example – keep pace with his intellectual, artistic, or physical success.

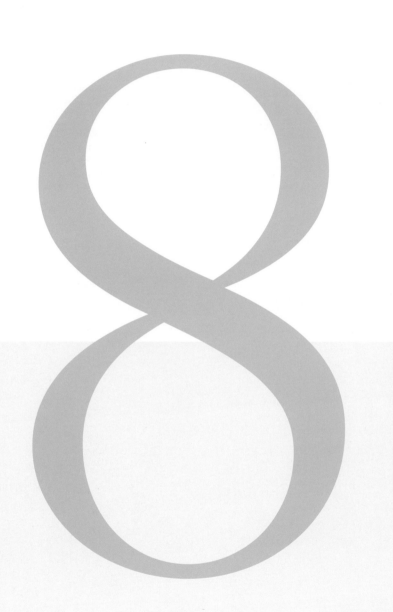
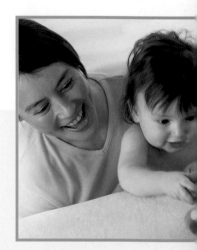

factors affecting development

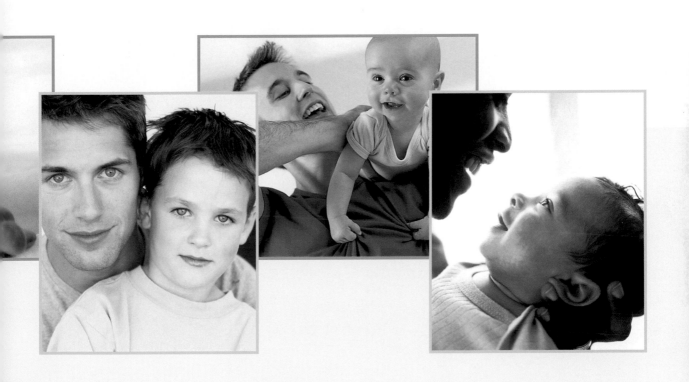

FACTORS AFFECTING DEVELOPMENT

Child development is rarely straightforward. So many factors play a part. There's what happens during the pregnancy and delivery, what skills and abilities your child is born with, and the way he is stimulated while raised at home, child care, and school. Heredity and environment interact to make your baby into a unique, special individual who has his own contribution to make to the world.

This chapter takes you through some of the key influences on your child's development – such as his genetic inheritance, family structure, his basic resilience to stress, his health, and your attitude as a parent. The more you are aware of factors impacting his development, the more you can play an active part in enabling him to fulfill his true potential.

Heredity

One of the delights of parenting is that you watch your child grow and develop. And it's only natural for you to want to know how much of your child's personality, abilities, behavior, and achievements are due to your skills as a parent and how much is due to inherited factors. This is what psychologists call "nature versus nurture," namely to what extent child development is caused by inherited qualities and to what extent it is due to environmental factors.

You probably delight in seeing that some of your child's physical characteristics, such as facial appearance, eye coloring, and build, have been passed genetically from you to him but you may be unaware that some of your psychological characteristics also may have passed to him. Although there is no definite proof, there is increasing evidence from scientific research that points to genetic influence being very important to the development of a child's personality.

Likelihood, not certainty

Even though research proves there is a genetic component to some aspects of child behavior, that doesn't mean the environment has no part to play. There are two important concepts for you to consider:

* **Genotype**: This is all the genetic material your child is born with. It is the blueprint of his development, and largely determines his potential characteristics and abilities. The genotype contains the information that, for instance, determines your child's eye color, what his eventual height is likely to be, and even when his second set of teeth are likely to appear.

Most psychologists acknowledge that it also contains some information about important

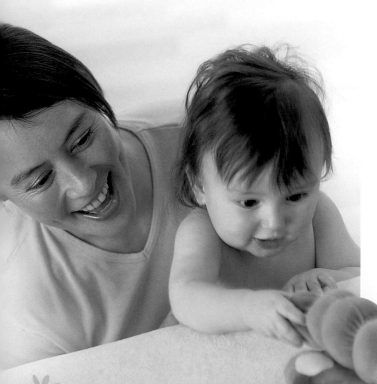

psychological traits as well, such as personality and temperament.

❋ *Phenotype:* This is the way all the genetic information in the genotype unfolds. The fact that a child has, for instance, the genetic potential to grow to a certain height doesn't mean that he definitely will – poor nutrition or chronic illness could result in a reduced rate of growth. The phenotype, therefore, is the outcome of the blueprint. Yet in the same way that a seed has the genetic potential to grow into a plant but can't achieve that outcome without adequate water and light, a child's growth and development are affected by other factors such as upbringing and environment.

Genes in perspective

The exact role of inherited abilities and characteristics remains unclear. While it is generally accepted that there is a significant genetic influence on development, there is also no doubt that the environment continues to play a huge part in your child's development. Inherited traits are not the whole explanation. Indeed, it is the interaction of your child's "nature" with the way you "nurture" him that eventually makes him a unique and wonderful individual. Your contribution to his life starts at conception and continues throughout his entire upbringing.

Personality

A child's personality can have a lot of bearing on the age at which she learns various skills. A baby who is independent, for example, may be eager to practice skills and may feed herself earlier and be toilet trained sooner than a more timid child. Similarly, if your child has a great desire to speak, she will probably do so before some of her other peers. From an early age, your child's personality has three

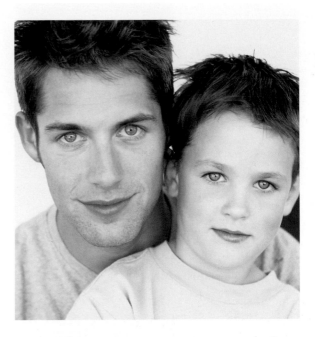

Peas in a pod
You can easily see the physical resemblance between this child and his father, but aspects of his personality and character may also have been inherited from his dad.

components, which can be examined on a continuum.

The first is emotional makeup. This is how she reacts to things, whether she becomes upset or distressed easily and intensely or whether she remains calm and easygoing.

Second, there is activity – how much effort does your baby put into doing things. Does she walk and talk quickly or slowly?

Finally, there is sociability. Does your child like to be with others and to share activities or is she more independent?

The process of development is very individual. Strive to adjust your parenting skills to ensure your child receives the level of reassurance, support, guidance, and help that will ensure she reaches her full potential.

Environmental influence

You previously read about the influence of genes on your child's development. But that isn't the whole story; there are some features of growth during the early years that can't be solely explained this way.

For instance, it is true that as children develop language they progress through the same stages in the same order at roughly the same age – an infant child will babble around eight months, say his first word around one year, and start to combine two words together to make a phrase around 18 months. If he is raised in a house where English is the only language spoken, he will speak in English; if he lives in a house where French is the only language spoken, he will learn to speak French, and so on. Environmental influences work in combination with genetic potential. Similarly, a child who is taught songs and nursery rhymes by his parents may be able to sing more songs and recite more rhymes than a child who has never heard them before.

The impact on heredity

The link between heredity and environment works in other subtle ways, too. They may be passively connected and related to the way parents organize their home life according to their needs and interests. For example, parents who enjoy music may play music throughout the day, may encourage their child to take music lessons, and may have musical instruments in the house. Not only does their child perhaps inherit musical tendencies that might make him more interested in music, but he also is raised in a musically-orientated environment, which allows his genetic predisposition to develop more readily.

Heredity and the environment also may have an active connection. A child naturally searches for an environment that allows him to express his genetic tendencies. That's why, for example, a child who is shy will probably avoid parties, preferring to stay at home and play on his own; he instinctively finds an environment that is right for his needs. Likewise, a child who is athletic may play for longer at activities that allow him to express his physical skills than at activities that are more sedentary. He intuitively finds an environmental niche, which allows him to develop in ways he wants.

Aiding your child's progress

Your baby is the wonderful individual that he is, partly through "nature" (because he has inherited a

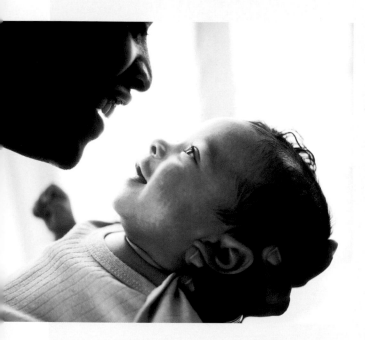

Not a blank slate
Personality traits may be obvious from birth if you know what to look for. They are demonstrated by a baby's general disposition – is she generally contented or usually irritable – and in the way she does things – is she awake and active most of the day or does she sleep for long periods and is generally easygoing when awake.

great deal from you and your partner) and partly through "nurture" (because he acquires a great deal through experience being raised by you and your partner). Nobody can say for sure which makes a more significant contribution to his development but the tips in the Positive Parenting box on the following page may enhance your parenting skills.

Be aware that your child's development is not entirely fixed and that nothing is inevitable. He is born with certain characteristics, skills, and abilities that can change depending on the way you raise him. He can also develop new characteristics, skills, and abilities as he grows.

Most importantly, every child has emotional needs as well as physical needs; for instance, he needs to be loved, to be valued, and to feel safe. A child who is denied love during the early years may actually have a slower rate of development. Just loving your child is a huge boost to his progress.

Prematurity

A premature baby is one who is born before the 37th week of pregnancy. Since a normal pregnancy lasts for approximately 40 weeks, a preterm baby arrives in this world less mature physically because her organs have not had as much time as they need to grow and prepare her for life outside the uterus. Premature babies born before 32 weeks of a pregnancy are particularly vulnerable and will typically require additional care and stimulation, at least in the early stages and often much longer. Although premature babies face a difficult start in life, research suggests less than one in 20 has significant long-term developmental problems.

Sensory stimulation

All babies need sensory stimulation in order to develop and grow to their fullest potential. Using all of your baby's senses, including auditory, visual, movement, and touch, you can enhance his understanding and thinking skills. Those activities that seem to work best emphasize gentle touch and movement and usually will enhance most aspects of your baby's development. But premature babies may be extrasensitive to light, sound, and touch for several months. Even playful conversation may be too intense for them and cause them to become fussy and look away. So parents should pay close attention to their infant's likes and dislikes. If too much is happening for her, take a break and resume the activity later.

Developing an emotional bond

The emotional attachment between parents and a premature baby may initially be a challenge because the baby may be kept in an incubator (an enclosed bed), which makes physical contact difficult. Even if you can't hold your baby, you may be able to touch her through the portholes of the enclosed bed. Spend as much time with her as possible, talking to her and letting her know that you are there.

Some people also tend to react in overcautious ways to a premature baby. For example, a research study showed a short film of a five-month-old baby to parents. If the parents were told that this baby was born prematurely, they displayed greater stress reactions when they heard the baby cry compared to other groups of parents who had been told the baby was born normally.

Other researchers have found a phenomenon known as "premature stereotyping," in which parents of premature babies still view their babies differently long after any developmental differences

POSITIVE PARENTING

Here are ways to help bring out your child's best.

Help your child feel confident

Expect your child to achieve. Your behavior toward him influences the way he views himself; if he believes you have confidence in his ability to, say, learn to ride a tricycle, then he will try a little harder because he starts to believe in himself, too. Low expectations may lead to underachievement.

Instead of thinking "that is just the way he is, he can't help himself," take a more positive view of your child. Tell yourself that there are always possibilities for change and progress, and that your child should be given every opportunity to develop his potential to the maximum. You and he never know what he could achieve until he tries.

Treat each child as special and unique

While your child may inherit some similar characteristics from you, he remains an individual. You can help him develop his full potential by recognizing his individual strengths and weaknesses and by supporting him according to his individual needs.

Be a good role model

Similarities between your behavior and that of your child's aren't only due to inherited factors. Given that your child lives with you, watches you, copies you, and is heavily affected by you, it is hardly surprising that he starts to behave like you. As a parent, you are your child's best role model. Therefore, take responsibility for any behavior that does not promote your child's well-being and, if necessary, work to change it.

between them and other babies the same age have disappeared.

Following advice from your neonatologist and pediatrician, you should have gentle, loving, physical contact with your baby whenever you can. This will help strengthen the bond between you. Have confidence in yourself and in your baby. Even though she was born early, like any other infant, she has the same emotional need to be loved.

Health and disability

A strong connection exists between your child's behavior and his health. Even a child who is usually very easy to be with can become irritable and uncooperative when sick – in fact, one of the signs of recovery will be that he is in better spirits, happier, and ready to play with his toys again or see his friends. When your child is ill, you may find that it takes a toll on you and other caregivers. You may need to miss work and stay up at night nurturing him back to good health and emotional stability.

Two additional psychological factors operate when your child experiences illness. The first is that your natural instinct as a parent when you see him sick and vulnerable is to cuddle and protect him. You will do anything you can medically and psychologically to restore him to good health. While that is part of your role as a parent, you should try to strike a balance between sensibly protecting your child and unnecessarily stifling him.

Understandably, your child likes you fussing over him when he is sick; that extra attention you give him makes him feel good; those special presents you may buy to cheer him up are very effective. And he'll want this to continue. So before he adapts and readjusts to being well again, you may find there are behavior difficulties such as a tantrum when it is time for you to leave him during the day again.

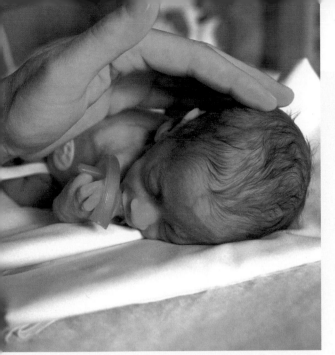

A loving touch
It is particularly important for premature babies to receive stimulation that imparts pleasurable sensations, though this needs to be gentle.

Strategies for managing illness

As soon as your child starts to recover, begin to return his life to normal. Make sure he is getting adequate sleep and encourage him to resume his previous daily routines, like getting out of bed for meals, sitting up to play with his toys, coloring at the kitchen table, or reading a book. Gradually draw him back into his regular life at home. Get him involved, slowly but steadily. Make sure, however, he does not push himself too far when he is not ready (although most children are good at regulating the pace of their recovery from a bout of illness).

Think carefully and discuss with other caregivers how you would like to manage his activities now that he is feeling better. Your child's natural tendency is to be on the go, to stay active, and to seek stimulation wherever he can find it. Illness only blocks that instinctive drive temporarily. The moment he starts to feel better, he will want to be up and about, so let him. Don't hold him back unnecessarily.

Impact of disability

All children have the same basic emotional and physical needs, but some children require additional help and support, perhaps arising from a physical, learning, or sensory disability. In addition, different family lifestyles, values, resources, parental interaction, and expectations also play an important part. Parents of a child with disability may face additional stresses, ranging from having to spend substantial dollars on special equipment and time on attending specialist appointments, to ensuring that the needs of other children in the family are adequately met, to blaming themselves for their child's disability.

Managing disability

Because no one can say for certain exactly how an infant with a disability will have developed by the time he is 5, 10, or 15 years old, you will need to accept some uncertainty about your child's future development. Understandably, this can be very challenging. It helps to concentrate on his individuality; he is a child who, along with having many other characteristics, traits, and abilities, also has a disability. See beyond his disability and relate to him as an individual. Focus on his strengths, not just on his challenges.

Make every effort you can to learn about your child's disability. Remember to seek trusted sources of information and ask your pediatrician if you have any questions or concerns. The website for the American Academy of Pediatrics (www.aap.org) is a good starting point. You may learn by talking to professionals connected with your child. You also may benefit from listening to the experiences of other parents and caregivers and from sharing your ideas with them.

It is important to know about the range of options available for a child with a disability. The Individuals with Disabilities Education Act (IDEA) is a federal law that requires states to develop special education programs for children with developmental disabilities. If your child is younger than three years, your pediatrician may refer him to an Early Intervention Program for services. If he is older than three at the time of the concern, the referral may be to your local public school.

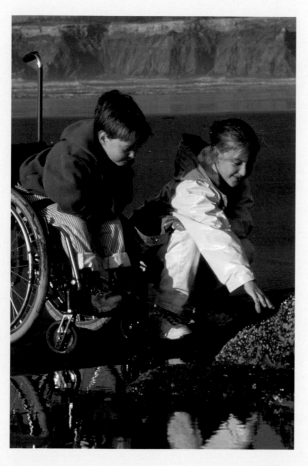

Parenting styles

What you think about parenting, your attitudes toward the way you believe your child should be raised, and your expectations of her – and of yourself – have a profound effect on your child's progress and development and your parenting behavior. Psychologists highlight four main parenting attitudes.

Authoritarian parents are likely to overcontrol and regulate their child's behavior; they expect and demand complete compliance to all their instructions and may react instantly when the rules are broken. Punishments for misbehavior are more frequent than rewards for good behavior. Caring words and physical contact with their children may not be displayed as often. Children of authoritarian parents may develop only adequate social skills and remain dependent on their parents.

In almost complete contrast to the authoritarian style, permissive parents are very relaxed about rules governing their children's behavior. They allow a child to do more or less as she pleases, and she is able to set her own limits for basic activities such as bedtime, meals, and leisure activities. Permissive parents are usually warm and affectionate in their relationship with their child. Children of permissive parents may have greater difficulty regulating their behavior.

Authoritative parents care very much about their child and her behavior, but want the child to take responsibility for managing her own behavior. By giving explanations for family rules, by encouraging

Focus on strengths
Learn all you can about your child's disability, but try to focus and build on his unique strengths as an individual. Nurturing these will help both of you through the challenges of disability.

the child to think about the consequences of her actions, and by using rewards more than punishments, authoritative parents develop a warm, supportive connection with their child. Children of authoritative parents tend to be self-reliant and socially confident.

Parents with an uninvolved approach to bringing up their child, either because of personal beliefs or personal stresses, may lack self-confidence in themselves as parents and may feel distant from their child. Children of parents who are uninvolved may have problems adjusting to life both at school and in social situations.

There are many factors that can play a role in weakening the attachment between a parent and child. If you feel like something is interfering with your involvement in your child's life, ask your physician to refer you to a mental health professional for further assistance.

Being a "good" parent

It's important to have the confidence to do what you think is right when it comes to raising your child. That said, if a spouse or significant other is involved in raising your child, you should discuss parenting tactics and agree on an approach. Consistency is key from all caregivers. There is nothing wrong with hearing perspectives about parenting from other people, but don't be afraid to do what you and your partner think is best for your child. Trust your judgment even though others might disagree. Every parent makes a mistake sometimes, that's simply part of the learning process. If you think you've done something wrong, resist the temptation to shower yourself with blame and guilt. See the event as an opportunity to learn. Don't be afraid to ask for help, support, or advice from family, friends, or a trained professional.

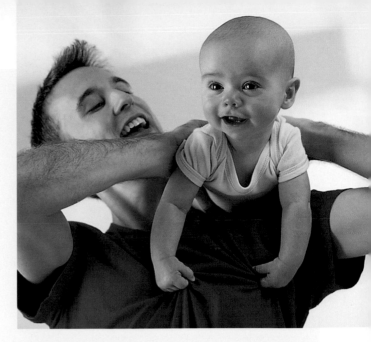

Projecting a positive attitude
Make being with your child a positive experience by rewarding all his efforts appropriately. Smiles and cuddles with let a baby know how pleased you are with him.

Just as you are different from your own parents, think of your child as an individual with her own collection of talents and traits; there is no point in comparing her with other children all the time (nor is there any point in comparing yourself with other parents). Be pleased with your child's individuality, and encourage her particular abilities.

Your child will gradually move forward at her own rate, whether it is that she is able to pull herself into a sitting position or that she can now solve the puzzle toy that she struggled with yesterday. Naturally, you have an idealized view of how you would like to be as a parent and how you would like your child to evolve. Hopefully these aspirations will be achieved to some extent, but don't demand too much of you or your child. Be proud of the wonderful developmental achievements – small or large – and let your child see that you are delighted with her.

Spoiling

Most people know what is meant by spoiling, yet it is hard to define. It's not just about giving your child lots of presents, nor is it simply letting her have what she wants, nor is it just giving in to her when she cries, pouts, or makes a fuss. Spoiling is less about how much your child is given and more about the way things are given and about the reasons why. The crucial factor is the balance of power between you and your child. If your child can twist you around her little finger, she may be spoiled.

Parents who spoil their child often confirm they do this out of love and good intentions. In some cases, parents may feel guilty that they work long hours and don't have enough time with their kids. They want the short amount of family time they have to be pleasant and they may do whatever it takes to avoid an argument or conflict. They may not even realize they are spoiling their child until someone else points it out to them.

So try not to give in to your child's demands all the time. Figuring out what your child needs versus what she wants is part of being a good parent. Be clear about what is acceptable behavior. Setting consistent guidelines will help reduce her need to test limits. Also, encourage your child to consider other people's feelings. Teach your child how to reach a compromise. For instance, if she wants to keep a ball all to herself, let her play with it for a few minutes, then give it to her brother or sister for the next few minutes.

Birth order

Whether your child is firstborn, second-born, or later-born, a middle-child or an only child, may influence to some extent the development of his personality and behavior. Some parents might feel it is important to treat each child the same way. But treating your children differently does not mean you are playing favorites. Treating each child as an individual is the best way to show that you appreciate how special he is.

Family size

There are many factors that may influence your decisions about the size of your family, such as personal preference, your own childhood experiences, health considerations, and financial constraints. It's up to you to decide how large or small you want it to be.

Age gap

Your child's place in the family is more than just his birth order and the number of his brothers and sisters, however – it also includes the age gap between siblings.

Children who are less than two years apart often have more conflict than siblings who are spaced further apart. This may be due to their competing over the same "turf." This might be something to keep in mind when planning a family. However, the effects of age gap on child development and each individual child's temperament are hard to predict and, therefore, you shouldn't base your plans for your family on this dimension alone. Also, relationships between siblings change and evolve as they grow older. The best time to think about having a second (or third or fourth, etc.) child is when you feel physically, emotionally, and financially ready for the experience and for the increase in your family size.

Blended families

With divorce, remarriage, and new living arrangements, children who barely knew each other may all of a sudden be forced to share space and their parents' time. At the same time, children are trying to get used to their parent's new marriage, a new stepparent and new stepsiblings. All of this can create conflict and rivalry between stepsiblings.

Whenever possible, it helps to give stepsiblings their own bedrooms. If they have to share a bedroom, allow each to have her own space, toys, and possessions. Do not expect stepsiblings to spend all of their time together. Make sure each child has time alone with her own parent. In addition, set aside time for family activities that everyone enjoys. Both parents should be involved in parenting and making decisions regarding each child.

If you and your new spouse decide to have another child, be open and honest with your other children. Involve them in planning for the new baby as much as possible. Reassure them that

First, middle, or last born?
Your child's place in your family may strongly influence her personality and character and is one of the ways in which your child demonstrates her uniqueness.

having a new baby does not mean that you will love them less.

Gender

Your child's sense of "boyness" and "girlness" (gender identity) develops throughout the early years of his or her life.

The true cause of gender differences is unknown. The "nature" explanation rests on biological evidence. For instance, research has revealed that from birth – and even during pregnancy itself – boys have a higher level of testosterone, which is linked to aggression and activity. It's hard to deny that this could play a part in determining gender differences. Similarly, the "nature" explanation also claims that since women are the only sex physically equipped to bear children, they must have a biological instinct to be caring and domesticated; and since men have to protect and feed their families, they must have a biological instinct to be aggressive. This theory is used to explain why

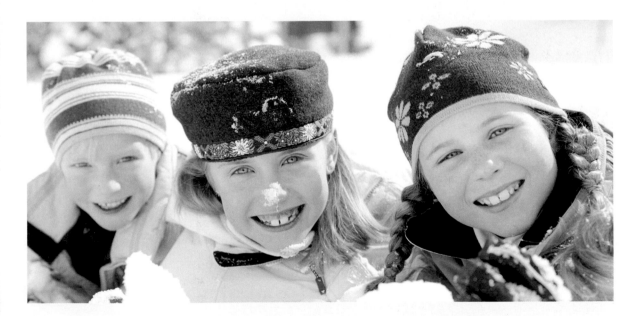

Your child's understanding of divorce, and the way he emotionally reacts to it, depends on many factors such as his age, temperament, and family support. The following are ways your child may react to a separation or divorce. Talk to your child's pediatrician if any of these behaviors become excessive or worrisome.

Under 3 years: Most children this age may be sad and not want to be separated from one parent. A child may have problems eating or sleeping, or show irritability or increased crying.

At 3–5 years: A child may have tantrums, become more clingy, or have problems with eating or sleeping. At this age, children often blame themselves for the divorce.

boys enjoy aggressive play while girls like playing with dolls.

In contrast, the "nurture" explanation of gender differences claims that parents react differently to boys and girls from the start and, therefore, create sex differences. Research studies have found, for example, that parents tolerate higher levels of aggression from boys than they do from girls, and that parents show more interest in their child's play when it involves toys normally associated with that gender. Almost certainly, however, these gender differences arise through an interaction of both nature and nurture.

The important point to remember is to offer your child a wide variety of play opportunities and experiences that support the development of many different skills.

Brothers and sisters

Your children's relationships with each other are influenced to some extent by gender and age, for instance, whether they are brother and sister or the same gender, or an older boy and a younger girl or older girl and younger boy. Many parents find that children of different genders seem to get along better

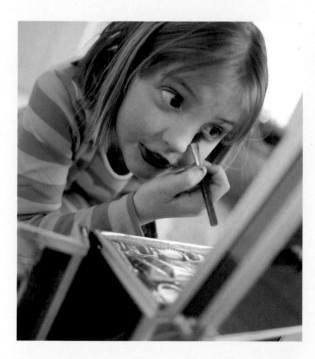

In the genes?
Toddlers of both sexes generally enjoy the same types of toys and activities, but over time they begin to identify themselves as masculine or feminine by associating with and mimicking the family members of their own sex.

with one another than do children of the same gender. A child's individual temperament as well as experiences within the family and relationships of a parent with their own siblings may play a role.

Your attitudes toward gender influence your children's attitudes, too. So if you assume that girls should sit quietly and play with dolls and that boys should be encouraged to be high-spirited and outgoing, then don't be surprised when your daughter frequently complains that her brother constantly pushes her around. It is important to teach all of your children, regardless of gender, to respect and support their siblings both at home and in the activities they choose.

Divorce and separation

Each year, more than one million children in the United States experience the divorce of their parents. The average divorce happens within the first seven years of a marriage, so many children are under the age of six. When divorce occurs, children need the support, patience, and love of both parents to help them through the experience.

Setting aside your differences

Every child wants to maintain a good relationship with mom and dad, whether they live with their parents or not. Staying together "for the sake of the children," however, is not always the best approach to managing parental disputes. When parents divorce, they must work together to help make the changes as easy as possible for the entire family. Parents can help by not forcing their children to take sides. Do not involve them in arguments between the two of you and do not criticize each other in front of your children.

POSITIVE PARENTING

There are a number of ways that parents can support their child through a family divorce.

Encourage her talk to you

If your child is around four or five years or older, she will have a good idea of what is going on. Explain the divorce in simple terms.

Listen to her fears

Aside from worrying about you, your child is also concerned about herself, the effects of the break-up on her home, her school, and her friends. Listen to her fears, treat them seriously, and reply honestly.

Keep to routines

The less your child's life is disrupted during and after a divorce or separation, the better. Changes of school, friends, activities, and daily routines should be kept to a minimum.

Take responsibility

Make sure your child understands that she had nothing to do with the divorce, that it was not her fault in any way. Let her know you love her and will not leave her.

Adhere to custody arrangements

Do what you can to sensibly agree on custody arrangements with your former partner and stick to whatever you've agreed. If you are having trouble with custody agreements, consider contacting a mediator for assistance.

Need for reassurance

Every child is different and reacts in her own way to a separation or divorce. But whatever her age, living through the experience is a stressful time. Her life at home is turned upside down, she misses the absent parent, she worries what will happen to her, and she probably is concerned that somehow the separation or divorce was her fault.

She needs lots of reassurance from both parents that she will be safe and that they will both continue to love her and to look after her.

Parents may be tempted to give their child false hope that they may get back together again (when they have no intention whatsoever of that happening) in order to make her feel more secure. That's a very risky strategy that may result in even further distress. Remember to be open and honest about the circumstances.

Stress

You are not the only one who feels stressed sometimes – your child can feel stressed, too. Your child experiences stress when he thinks that the demands he faces exceed his capability, in other words, when he finds himself in distressing situations beyond his control – it's that feeling of pressure, which results in worry, tension, sadness, and even anger.

There are many different ways that stress can show in your child's behavior. For instance, a normally easygoing child could become irritable and uncooperative, his eating and sleeping habits could become erratic, and he might be overly worried about things that normally don't bother him. A child in school may start having learning difficulties as well as behavioral issues with his classmates. An independent child may become more needy of one or both parents. In some cases, an older child who is

POSITIVE PARENTING

You can help your child to avoid stressful situations or, when unavoidable, to cope with them better.

Listen to your child's concerns

They may appear trivial to you but they are very real to him, otherwise he wouldn't be so upset. He will feel less stressed just from having you listen to him and treat him respectfully. Try hard to have a relaxed, communicative relationship with your child, so that he feels able to discuss any concerns with you at any time.

Discourage negative self-talk

Take an optimistic approach and always value effort as well as achievement. Whenever you hear your child make disparaging or negative statements about himself and his skills, point out that he has lots of strong points, too. Identify your child's strengths and unique interests and try to nurture them.

Teach him some stress-reducing skills

When he becomes stressed because he faces what appears to be an overwhelming task (for instance, cleaning his room), show him how to do this in small steps. Also, an impending challenge will be less stressful if your child prepares for it in advance. Before singing to others in preschool, for instance, he could rehearse his song with you.

Intervene early

Your child is probably most stressed by events that he does not have time to prepare for. Giving him advance warning allows him to get ready in plenty of time. Help him tackle problems when they first arise, rather than leaving them until the last minute.

very stressed may behave as if
he is much younger, for instance, he might start
to suck his thumb. Often, a regression in your
child's behavior is the most likely sign of his
being under stress.

Common causes

Every child reacts uniquely to life events, and
therefore it cannot be said with certainty that every
child will have the same responses. Many causes of
stress in childhood are linked to family and friends.
For instance, parental separation causes stress for the
children involved, or a child could be stressed by
pressure from his siblings, or because he feels he isn't
able to make friends at school. Other causes of stress
could include health, developmental, or learning
challenges. Remember to seek help as needed to
support your child through stressful times.

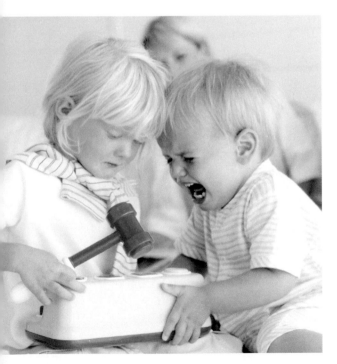

In the know... *Childhood stresses*

*Stress is hard to measure because it is very
personal – what one child perceives as stressful (for
instance, an amusement park ride), his friend could
easily perceive as exciting. Some children experience
stress to such an extent that it has an adverse effect
on their lives. Some children are more susceptible to
stress than others. When a young child is under
stress, he may act out, withdraw, or regress (such
as start thumb sucking again). Help your child
through stressful times by listening and by
providing support.*

Resilience

It is well established that children thrive best in a
stable, nurturing family environment. In contrast, a
child who experiences stresses such as parental
divorce, emotional neglect, lack of housing,
frequent changes in child care or school, or
inconsistent discipline at home, are more prone to
behavioral and psychological difficulties. But there
are many children who experience these same
stresses and who still achieve satisfactory
development in spite of them. Psychologists describe
these children as "resilient"; they are able to cope
with life's adverse circumstances and come through
generally unaffected.

Sibling rivalry
Tension between siblings is common. However, if a strongly-
willed child is always allowed to have his own way, it may
have a negative effect on more even-tempered siblings as well
as the family as a whole.

All children will experience stressful times at some point in their lives. Parents can make a big difference in preparing their children to be able to meet and overcome those challenges.

Characteristics of a resilient child

A resilient child is likely to be socially confident, able to get along well with both other children and adults, and readily communicates her thoughts and feelings.

A resilient child may also be solution-focused. That is why, when confronted with a problem, she is able to think of a way around it, or find a solution. Rather than feeling overwhelmed by the challenge, she uses her resources to effect change.

Building resilience
A broad range of play opportunities, both free and structured, can help build resilience.

A child is more resilient to pressure when she is independent – able to stand on her own two feet, when she can think and act for herself, and when she feels she can exercise some control on the world around her. If she is optimistic, she can concentrate more on the positives of a situation than the negatives. She doesn't pretend there are no hurdles to climb, she just has the self-belief that she has what it takes to climb them. Her determination drives her to persist until she achieves success.

Reducing your child's vulnerability

Parents who are emotionally warm, caring, and loving, create a psychological bond that can help their child deal with future stress. A connection with at least one loving adult is vitally important. In addition, a supportive and inclusive community, at home or school, can also play a role. It also helps to have high expectations of your child. Don't push her

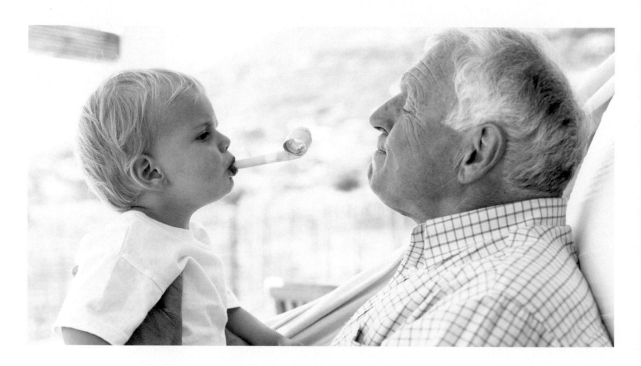

too hard or demand too much from her; just want her to do her best and encourage her to aim high because you are confident she has the ability.

When you hold your child to high expectations it means much more than encouraging her to perform well or produce successfully. It means you know that she is a good person inside, and that you cherish that essential goodness and expect it to show. Even when she misbehaves you never stray from the firmly held knowledge that she is essentially a kind, caring person. She will learn to see herself as a good person.

Behavior concerns

There could be times when your child's behavior is so challenging, so demanding, or so troubling, that you worry about its long-term impact. Ask yourself the following questions:

How long has her behavior been like this? If you have only noticed her troubled behavior over the past few weeks, then the chances are this is temporary and will resolve.

What is the effect of her troubled behavior? If it only happens with you, but not with others, you can worry less about it. However, it is more serious if all those around her complain to you, or if her behavior is causing problems with her friends and siblings.

What have you tried to do to help? Serious troubled behavior may continue when efforts to improve it have failed. If you have made considerable efforts to improve your child's behavior, to resolve her difficulties, but they still persist, the problem is probably more serious and needs discussing with your child's pediatrician.

POSITIVE PARENTING

You can help your child become more resilient in the following ways.

Offer support, not confrontation

Although your child's behavior may be difficult to manage, look for ways to help her rather than battling with her. Try to understand the world from your child's point of view. Her anger may seem unjustified, but it will help if you listen to her side of the story. Talking together reduces stress.

Reward the positives

Catch your child doing something good (no matter how small) and praise her or reward her with a sign of affection, a sticker, or a star on a chart.

Think how you might change

Consider what possible changes you might make in your own behavior toward your child, which could, in turn, make a difference in her behavior.

Set reasonable targets

Your child's difficult behavior isn't going to change overnight; it will take time. Set attainable goals, and show your delight when she reaches them.

Don't give all the answers

A resilient child gains confidence after she grows to trust her own competence. She does this when she learns that she is capable of making wise decisions and figuring out how to handle difficult situations. Be available to be a sounding board and to offer guidance when it is requested. Sometimes, though, the best thing to do is "get out of the way" (after assuring safety) and let your child trust her own abilities.

GROWTH CHARTS

At every complete physical exam your child will have his height and weight measured and plotted on a growth chart similar to those found on the following pages. For infants, a head circumference measurement will also be taken (see page 218). Starting at two years of age your child's Body Mass Index (BMI) should be calculated and plotted. BMI is a ratio of your child's weight in relation to his height. If you have any questions about your child's growth, speak to your pediatrician.

BOYS LENGTH/WEIGHT BIRTH TO 36 MONTHS   BOYS LENGTH/WEIGHT 2 TO 20 YEARS

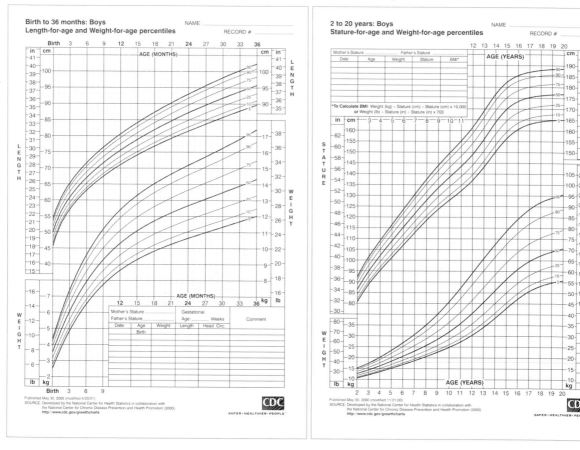

GIRLS LENGTH/WEIGHT BIRTH TO 36 MONTHS

GIRLS LENGTH/WEIGHT 2 TO 20 YEARS

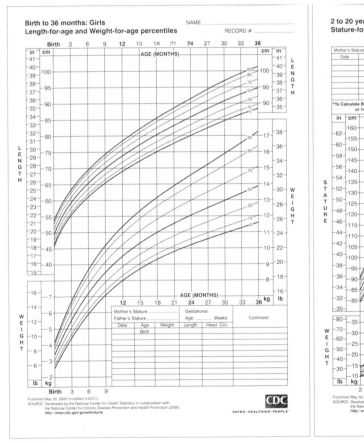

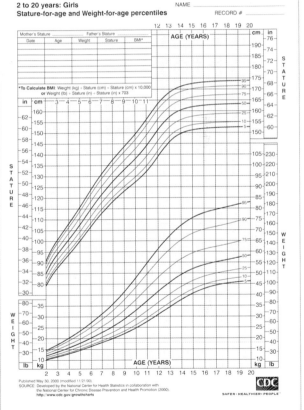

BOYS HEAD CIRCUMFERENCE

GIRLS HEAD CIRCUMFERENCE

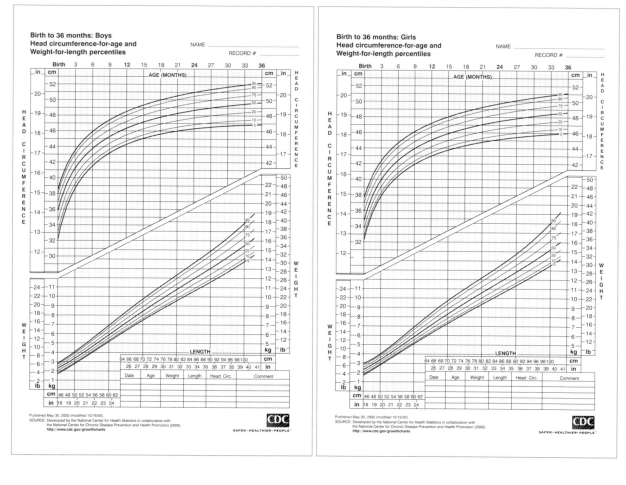

BOYS BODY MASS INDEX (BMI)

GIRLS BODY MASS INDEX (BMI)

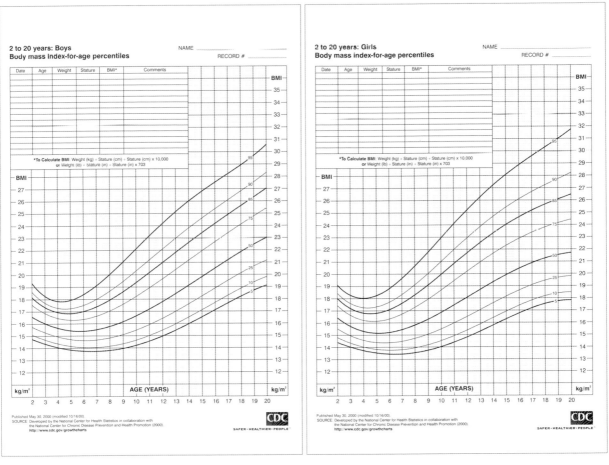

index

A

Accommodation, sight, 74
Active responses, 96
Activities
  to encourage bonding, 97
  to encourage learning,
    100
  to encourage sense of
    touch, 87
  see also Games
Age gap, 208
Aggressive behavior,
  143–147
Amblyopia, 187
Anger, 143–147
Art and Creative Materials
  Institute (ACMI), 165
Asperger syndrome,
  195–196
Attachment, 136–138
Attention Deficit
  Hyperactivity Disorder
  (ADHD), 191–195
Authoritarian parents, 206
Authoritative parents,
  206–207
Autism spectrum disorder
  (ASD), 195–196

B

Babbling, 103, 104, 110
Baby blues, 134
Baby games, 36
Baby language, 104
Baby massage, 87
Baby walkers, 32
Back to sleep campaign, 14
Balanced diet, 40, 116–117
Ball games, 41
Banging objects, 56
Bath play, 141
Bed-wetting, 178–179
Behavior concerns, 215
Benign Urinary Frequency,
  172

Bike riding, 40–41
Birth order, 208
Bladder, 171–172
  control, 168–170
Body language, 92, 101,
  105, 107
Body Mass Index (BMI), 216
Bonding, 71, 84, 96,
  133–135
  activities to encourage, 97
Books, 54, 88, 110
Bottle-feeding, 134
Bow legs, 25
Bowel, 173–174
  control, 168–170, 173
Brain, development of, 70
Breastfeeding, 21, 116, 134
Building skills, 60
Bullying, 147, 191

C

Caffeine, 117
Car seats, 19
Cerebral palsy, 32, 183,
  184, 188
Child centred environment,
  93
Choking, danger of, 66
Clapping hands, 53
Climbing, 33–35
Cochlear implant, 186
Cognitive ability, 98–100
Colic, 142
Coloboma, 187
Communication, 101–108,
  134
Concentration, 98
Constipation, 173–174
Convergence, sight, 74
Conversation, 112, 118
Coordinating objects, 56–57
Coordination, hand-eye, 44
Copying adults, 54
Counting games, 95
Craft activities and
  materials, 58

Crawling, 22–24
Crayons and paints, using,
  58, 62
Cross-modal transfer, 71
Cruising, 25–27
Crying, 102
Curiosity, 100, 114, 119
Cutting, 64
Cytomegalovirus (CMV),
  186

D

Depression, 193
  postpartum, 134
Developmental delay, 182
Diabetes mellitus, 179
Diarrhea, 174
Disability, 205–206
Disruptive behavior,
  189–191
Distance perception, 76
Divergence, sight, 74
Divorce and separation,
  208, 211
  age and reactions to, 210
  supporting the child
    through, 211
Down syndrome, 184
Drawing, 62–64
Dressing, 65–67
  parental participation, 67
Dressing up, 58, 67
Drinking, 66
Dropping and putting
  down, 52
Dyslexia, 188

E

EIGHT MONTHS
attachment, 136
crawling, 23
mental development, 94
personality, 130
picking up and holding,
  49, 51

sense of touch, 87
sociability, 130
suitable toys, 88
turning over, 18
understanding language,
  113
EIGHTEEN MONTHS
attachment, 137
building with blocks, 60
communication skills,
  101
development of hearing,
  81
development of sight, 77
drinking from a cup, 66
feeding, 65
game play, 124
mental development, 94
personality, 130–131
sociability, 130–131
speech development, 109
suitable toys, 88
understanding language,
  113
using a pencil, 62
walking, 31
ELEVEN MONTHS
crawling, 23
feeding, 65
sense of touch, 87
sitting, 21
standing, 26
walking, 31
Emotional intelligence, 92
Emotions, 121, 139–141
Empathy, 157–160
Environment, effect on
  development, 202
Exercise, importance of, 40
Exercises, 36–37
Expressive language, 82

F

Face recognition, 71
Family size, 208
Fantasy play, 143

acknowledgments

American Academy of Pediatrics (AAP)

AAP Medical Editor-in-Chief
Tanya Remer Altmann, MD, FAAP

AAP Board of Directors Reviewer
Burton F. Willis, MD, FAAP

AAP Committee and Section Reviewers
Daniel G. Batton, MD, FAAP
Committee on Fetus and Newborn
William L. Coleman, MD, FAAP
Committee on Psychosocial Aspects of Child and Family Health
Kerry L. English, MD, FAAP
Committee on Early Childhood, Adoption and Dependent Care
Jorge E. Gomez, MD, FAAP
Council on Sports Medicine and Fitness
Frank R. Greer, MD, FAAP
Committee on Nutrition
Pamela C. High, MD, MS, FAAP
Committee on Early Childhood, Adoption and Dependent Care
Michelle M. Macias, MD, FAAP
Section on Developmental and Behavioral Pediatrics
Robert A. Saul, MD, FAAP
Section on Genetics and Birth Defects
Gary A. Smith, MD, DrPH , FAAP
Committee on Injury, Violence, and Poison Prevention
Dennis L. Vickers, MD, MPH, FAAP
Committee on Early Childhood, Adoption and Dependent Care
Robert G. Voigt, MD, FAAP
Section on Developmental and Behavioral Pediatrics

Additional Reviewers
Howard J. Bennett, MD, FAAP
Jenn Berman MFT, PsyD
Ari Brown, MD, FAAP
Kimberly Carlson MS, CCC-SLP

Heather A. Cornett, MD, FAAP
Howard Goldstine, MD, FAAP
Kenneth R. Ginsburg, MD, MS Ed, FAAP
Marilyn Greene, MFT
William Greene, MD, FAAP
Laura A. Jana, MD, FAAP
Robert Nudelman, MD, FAAP
Angelee K. Reiner, MD, FAAP
Kristin J. Santangelo, MD
David Scherr, MD, FAAP
Sloane Sevran, MD, FAAP
Leslie Spiegel, MD, FAAP

AAP Staff
Errol R. Alden, MD, FAAP
Executive Director/CEO
Roger F. Suchyta, MD, FAAP
Associate Executive Director
Maureen DeRosa, MPA
Director, Department of Marketing and Publications
Mark Grimes,
Director, Division of Product Development
Eileen Glasstetter, MS
Manager, Consumer Publishing
Holly Kaminski
Coordinator, Product Development

Picture Credits
Front Jacket (second from right) David Murray; page 6 Professor Stuart Campbell; page 19 Index Stock/Photolibrary; page 28 www.bloomingmarvellous.co.uk; page 37 (top right) Workbook/Photolibrary; pages 58–9 Getty Images; page 60 Getty Images; page 120 Aflo/Photolibrary; page 132 Anthea Sieveking/Wellcome Photo Library; page 149 (bottom) Photononstop/Photolibrary; page 150 Getty Images; page 152 Dynamic Graphics/Photolibrary; page 157 BSIP/Photolibrary; page 164 Getty Images; page 165 (top) Getty Images; page 166 BabyBjorn; page 168 photo@imagesprite.com; page 170 (top) BabyBjorn; page 172 Getty Images; page 176 (bottom) BabyBjorn; page 177 Mother and Baby Picture Library/Ian Hooton; page 191 BSIP/Photolibrary; page 205 Phototake/Photolibrary; page 206 Index Stock/Photolibrary; page 209 Workbook/Photolibrary; page 210 Workbook/Photolibrary